TRAINING FOR TWO

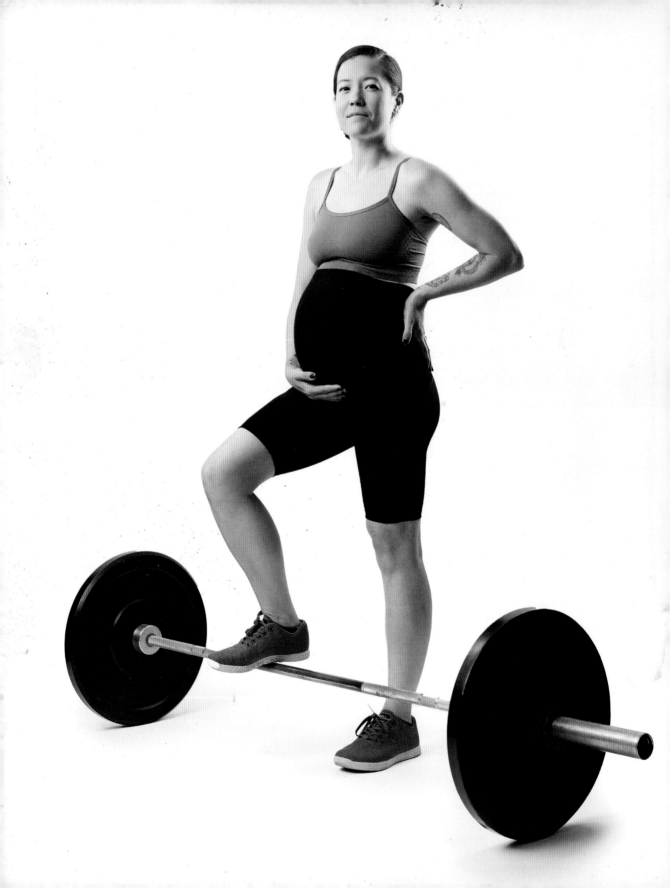

TRAINING
FOR TWO

Safe and Smart Prenatal Exercises
for a Smoother Pregnancy,
Easier Birth, and Healthier Newborn

GINA CONLEY, MS

FAIR WINDS

Quarto.com

First Published in 2024 by Fair Winds Press,
an imprint of The Quarto Group, 100 Cummings
Center, Suite 265-D, Beverly, MA 01915, USA.
T (978) 282-9590 F (978) 283-2742

Fair Winds Press titles are also available at discount
for retail, wholesale, promotional, and bulk purchase.
For details, contact the Special Sales Manager by email
at specialsales@quarto.com or by mail at The Quarto
Group, Attn: Special Sales Manager, 100 Cummings
Center, Suite 265-D, Beverly, MA 01915, USA.

28 27 26 25 24   1 2 3 4 5

ISBN: 978-0-7603-8754-2

Digital edition published in 2024
eISBN: 978-0-7603-8755-9

Library of Congress Cataloging-in-Publication Data
is available.

Design: Kelley Galbreath
Cover Image: Lisa Miyamoto, Makana Photography LLC
www.makana-photography.com
Page Layout: Kelley Galbreath
Photography: Lisa Miyamoto, Makana Photography LLC
www.makana-photography.com
Illustration: Alexandra Gordon www.alexandragordon.com

Printed in China

DEDICATION

FOR MY HUSBAND, BARRON.
Thank you for your support from the beginning.
All that I have been able to create has been thanks to you.
And for Adeline, my first child. Without the journey we
were on together, there would be no MamasteFit. Thank you
for my inspiration and for teaching me how to be a mom.

CONTENTS

FOREWORD

I'M FOREVER THANKFUL FOR MEETING GINA back in 2017. At that time, we were both new moms navigating our first postpartum experience.

We both were "rocked" by pregnancy, birth, and postpartum. For both of us, something just didn't line up with how "the system" was telling people to navigate exercise, training, and pain during pregnancy, birth, and postpartum.

At that time, Gina was still active duty in the military and starting up Mamaste-Fit. I was pivoting my whole identity as a sports medicine physical therapist and transitioning to the pelvic rehab world.

Gina and I both were starving for more information. We were scouring every book, continuing education course, and research article on pregnancy, birth, and pelvic health to better serve our small community in North Carolina.

In the "pregnancy" exercise section of most pregnancy books, they talk about yoga, walking, and Kegel exercises as ways to "safely" exercise in pregnancy. If you're lucky, you get some "core activation" or some "functional movement" like squats, but not always. As for managing things like common pregnancy discomforts? Pregnancy belts, braces, and the elimination of the offending movement(s) or "just wait until the baby comes" are the typical things recommended.

There is no discussion of the root cause or an understanding of the anatomy or physiology of the changes in pregnancy—only fear-based information that takes autonomy and activity away from the pregnant person instead of encouraging exercise and empowerment through information and evidence from research.

It was amazing to find a kindred spirit in Gina, who truly believed that pregnancy was not an illness and that the common symptoms of pregnancy were not to be ignored. Her hunger for information and drive to learn were so strong that she used all of her study and understanding of the anatomy and physiology of pregnancy, birth, and pelvic floor rehab to create programs that are incredibly powerful and effective.

All that said, the biggest blessing of all was meeting someone who believed so strongly in what she was creating that she couldn't help but start shouting this information from the rooftops—to spread this information from beyond our small town to the world. Gina knows, and feels deeply, that *everyone* deserves this information. Her curation of countless free blogs, social media posts, and resources has undoubtedly affected millions. Witnessing Gina in the relentless pursuit of changing the way we approach pregnancy has been completely awe-inspiring.

If you are looking for the most comprehensive and well-informed guide to a strong, confident, and bold pregnancy, look no further. While I know Gina will never be satisfied, and many, many more editions will come out in the years to follow as she continues her pursuit of more information, I can confidently say that you, right now, are holding the best resource for training through pregnancy ever created.

—*Hayley Kava PT, MPT, PRC*

INTRODUCTION

WELCOME TO *TRAINING FOR TWO*! If you're like me, you have no idea what to do with the endless onslaught of conflicting information about prenatal fitness. However, there is a consensus between the American College of Obstetricians and Gynecologists (ACOG), the Centers for Disease Control and Prevention (CDC), and other major governing bodies that exercise throughout pregnancy benefits you and your baby.

This book will guide you through approaching fitness during all three trimesters, but this book is much more than just "pregnancy-safe" exercises. This book is a collection of my experience as a perinatal fitness trainer and birth doula, and the expertise of a pelvic floor physical therapist and labor and delivery nurse who has offered support in the development of this book. After reading this book, you'll know which exercises to include in your prenatal fitness workouts to stay strong and remain comfortable (pain is not a requirement of pregnancy), while also preparing for birth and the postpartum period. You'll know why certain movement patterns are helpful and how to properly modify them based on your individual pregnancy. Plus, you'll learn how to move confidently through your birth and early postpartum.

During my first pregnancy, I felt clueless about the dos and don'ts of prenatal fitness. The abundance of conflicting advice and rigid rules about fitness was quite intimidating. Then, add on the severe nausea and overwhelming fatigue of my first trimester, and that derailed any plan I had to work out during that time.

As the second trimester arrived, I remained uncertain about the right approach to exercise. I was fearful of exercising, as most of the guidance for prenatal fitness was a long list of things to avoid. I found myself excessively modifying movements out of fear of harming my baby. I spent the remainder of my pregnancy fairly active, but I was mostly confused on what I should be doing. I also suffered from sacroiliac joint pain, also known as *pelvic girdle pain*, throughout the second half of my pregnancy, which made walking and exercising painful. I was given no solutions on how to manage this other than to see a chiropractor and wait for birth.

After my first pregnancy, I began my study on prenatal and postnatal fitness. I started my company, MamasteFit, and began coaching in-person clients during their pregnancy and postpartum phases, and then I began supporting births as a doula. Merging professional insights with my research, I designed comprehensive prenatal fitness programs. These programs aimed for not only a physically strong pregnancy but also a comfortable one, preparing clients for the demands of childbirth through exercises promoting pelvic opening and optimizing pelvic floor function.

Sadly, during my subsequent two pregnancies, I suffered pregnancy losses in the first trimester. An insensitive remark suggested that lifting weights and exercising might have caused my miscarriages. This comment deeply hurt me, insinuating I had endangered my babies, which was far from the truth. It's important to clarify that exercise does not trigger miscarriage, nor does it elevate the likelihood of prenatal complications. On the contrary, research has repeatedly demonstrated that engaging in physical activity is incredibly beneficial for both you and your baby, can reduce prenatal complications, and may improve birth outcomes—but more about that later.

After our losses, we fortunately had two successful pregnancies with our second and third children, with no complications. I capitalized on the prenatal fitness programs I'd developed to support my pregnancies and childbirth preparation. These subsequent pregnancies were markedly different than my first. I was more confident in moving my body throughout my pregnancy without fear of hurting myself or my baby. Thanks to preventive exercises promoting pelvic stability, the sacroiliac pain that I suffered in my first pregnancy was remarkably reduced. My understanding of pelvic mechanics and my use of exercises for pelvic opening and pelvic floor relaxation facilitated easier labor experiences. The information in this book can do the same for you.

Compiling my knowledge, I've crafted this book to empower you as you navigate your prenatal fitness journey. This book equips you to develop prenatal fitness programs that don't just foster strength but also alleviate pain and ensure prenatal comfort. Furthermore, you'll gain the tools to use your prenatal workouts to prepare for birth and the postnatal period.

The book starts by highlighting the benefits of prenatal fitness for both you and your baby. Next, it offers insights into approaching fitness during the prenatal period, followed by trimester-specific recommendations. Then, it delves deeply into leveraging prenatal fitness for birth readiness, encompassing exercises promoting pelvic opening and pelvic floor release, which will guide you on how to move through your labor. Finally, the book concludes with a focus on supporting your early postpartum recovery.

My hope is that this book instills in you the confidence and knowledge to engage in exercise throughout your pregnancy in a manner that positively affects your prenatal, birthing, and motherhood journey. Let's get started.

PART 1

WHY PRENATAL FITNESS? BENEFITS FOR YOU AND BABY

MOST OF US UNDERSTAND THAT EXERCISING throughout pregnancy is beneficial, and what we do (or don't do) during our pregnancy can affect our child's lifelong health. That is a lot of pressure! Then add on the endless flood of unsolicited advice from onlookers commenting on the safety (or danger, rather) of exercise during pregnancy. All of it is well-meaning advice attempting to protect your baby from you, which contributes to a feeling of uncertainty and affects your confidence. This uncertainty expands to almost every aspect of pregnancy.

Here's the thing: Though well-meaning, Aunt Linda and Random Sally are not up-to-date on the current research for prenatal fitness. There are a lot of benefits of exercising, encompassing lifting weights and vigorous exercise, for both you and your baby. Exercising throughout your pregnancy is generally safe; there are very few exercises that are inherently dangerous (and these are mostly due to the increased fall risk).

The American College of Obstetricians and Gynecologists (ACOG) recommends a minimum of 150 minutes of moderate-intensity exercise per week throughout pregnancy. ACOG even recommends resistance training throughout pregnancy. If exercise were unsafe, the governing body of obstetricians would not recommend it!

In the first part of this book, we will explore the advantages of engaging in prenatal fitness that benefit you and your baby. Understanding that your efforts can positively influence your baby's well-being might provide you with increased motivation. We will also break down common myths associated with prenatal fitness so you can feel confident approaching your workouts.

ONE
THE BENEFITS OF PRENATAL FITNESS FOR YOU

LET'S START BY DISCUSSING HOW prenatal fitness can benefit you during the prenatal and postpartum periods.

Pregnancy brings about physiological changes that affect virtually every system in your body, from cardiovascular and hormonal changes to musculoskeletal adjustments. These physiological adaptations (by which we mean the adaptations your body makes to accommodate a pregnancy) can be enhanced with exercise. Additionally, prenatal fitness helps alleviate common discomforts like lower back and pelvic pain, supporting a more comfortable pregnancy.

Another benefit is that exercising throughout pregnancy can reduce or delay the need for labor induction and birth interventions, increase the speed of labor and delivery, and decrease complications during birth. Prenatal fitness can also support an easier recovery from birth and reduce the prevalence of postpartum anxiety and depression. So let's dive into the physiological changes that take place throughout pregnancy, and the advantages fitness has for your pregnancy, birth, and postpartum recovery.

BENEFITS OF PRENATAL FITNESS FOR PREGNANCY

During pregnancy, your body undergoes changes that make it work better while it manages the stress of making a baby. This applies to virtually every system in your body. For example, your blood volume rises, aiding oxygen and nutrient distribution, improving waste removal, and boosting cooling and temperature control. The respiratory system enhances oxygen and carbon dioxide transfer at a cellular level, an effect that is completely unique to pregnancy. Your metabolism changes, prioritizing carbohydrates for the baby's energy by using other nutrients for your own. Overall, the pregnant body undergoes significant physiological shifts. In this section, we'll break down how each system changes and then describe how exercise can enhance these changes, ultimately benefiting both you and your baby.

THE CARDIOVASCULAR SYSTEM

The cardiovascular system improves significantly during pregnancy. Your cardiovascular system is responsible for:

- Transporting oxygen and nutrients throughout the body
- Removing metabolic waste
- Protecting against disease and infection
- Maintaining body temperature

Imagine the cardiovascular system as a complex network of roads (blood vessels) with vehicles (blood cells) transporting goods throughout a bustling city (your body). During pregnancy, the roads expand, accommodating more lanes (larger blood vessels), creating additional routes (increased capillaries), and allowing for a greater number of vehicles (higher blood volume). Consequently, your body becomes incredibly adept at transporting vital nutrients to both you and your baby. Remarkably, all of this occurs effortlessly on your end (apart from, you know, creating an entire human).

It should come as no surprise that exercise enhances the function of your cardiovascular system. That's how it works for nonpregnant people, after all. But during pregnancy, it goes a step further by actually amplifying the adaptations your body is already making. Prenatal exercise increases the number of roads and cars by increasing blood volume an additional 10 to 15 percent. It also accelerates the pace of these cars by increasing the volume of blood pumped with each heartbeat. Finally, exercise improves your body's ability to use the increased flow of oxygen and nutrients and more efficiently remove metabolic waste.

Improved cardiovascular fitness may also mitigate the risk of a Cesarean birth because of the increase in oxygen levels in the umbilical artery blood, consequently enhancing your baby's resilience to labor-related stress (more on this in chapter 2).

THE RESPIRATORY SYSTEM

The respiratory system is responsible for exchanging gases, specifically taking in oxygen and removing carbon dioxide. During pregnancy, there is an incredible change that occurs at the cellular level that improves how well you exchange these gases in your tiny air sacs. You can think of your lungs like an upside-down tree. Air enters the tree trunk (your trachea, or throat), and then flows through the branches (bronchi, or the branches of your lungs). The tree's branches continually split and get smaller until you reach the end of the branch, where a leaf (alveoli, or air sac) transfers oxygen and carbon dioxide to the tree.

Now imagine this tree (your respiratory system) has a conveyor belt that is transporting vital supplies. When you take a breath, air is drawn into your lungs, moving through these branches. This path ultimately leads to the tiny air sacs, the leaves.

Within the air sacs, changes in pressure facilitate the exchange of gases. During pregnancy, these pressure changes become more adept, ensuring a faster and more efficient exchange of oxygen into the bloodstream and the removal of carbon dioxide from it. It's like optimizing the speed and accuracy of the conveyor belt's operations to meet the growing oxygen demands. Pregnancy is the only time in our lives that our lungs get better at breathing at this cellular level!

EXTREME FATIGUE AND NAUSEA: A SYMPTOM OF LOW BLOOD PRESSURE

ONE OF THE MORE NOTICEABLE pregnancy symptoms is first-trimester fatigue and nausea, both of which are side effects of lower blood pressure. Imagine it like this: The number of lanes per road has suddenly doubled in size, but the number of cars has remained the same. This results in a decrease in the overall volume of vehicles to fill up this expanded roadway, leading to a drop in traffic density (blood pressure). This decrease in blood pressure can lead to feelings of fatigue and nausea.

In the second trimester, the blood volume finally catches up (there are enough cars on the road), and you feel more energized. Throughout pregnancy, your blood volume will increase by around 40 percent. That is a lot of new cars transporting goods all around your circulatory system.

Additionally, the hormone progesterone, which surges during pregnancy, plays a crucial role in these respiratory improvements. Progesterone stimulates an increase in both the depth and the rate of breathing. This means that each breath becomes more profound and more frequent, resulting in the ability to inhale up to 40 to 50 percent more air with every breath. It's as if more skilled workers have been added to the conveyor belt, working tirelessly to ensure a steady and efficient flow of oxygen to the bloodstream while swiftly removing carbon dioxide. While exercising during pregnancy does not improve this gas exchange, it does improve your ability to transport all this extra oxygen, and it improves your ability to do it more efficiently.

If you recall from the previous section, the cardiovascular system has all these extra side roads (capillaries) that make it easier to bring goods (oxygen and nutrients) to your cells. It's like having side roads that connect to a neighborhood—if there were no side roads that connected to the houses in the neighborhood, you would need to get out of your car on the highway and walk to deliver a package. This would increase the time it takes you to deliver a package. In comparison, if you could drive right up to a house to deliver a package, this would really expedite the delivery. This happens when you exercise—your body creates more side roads (capillaries) that bring you right up to the door of your cells to deliver oxygen and other vital nutrients and take away metabolic waste. Additionally, exercise increases the strength of the muscles that support breathing, making it easier to bring air into your lungs.

Now that you have all this extra oxygen, exercising makes you more efficient at using it and converting it into energy. When you exercise, you increase the number of mitochondria, your energy factories, in your cells. They take the oxygen you inhale and convert it into usable energy for your body. A larger number of mitochondria improves your muscular strength, boosts your endurance, and increases your aerobic capacity, or the maximum amount of oxygen that your body can use during exercise. Think of it as having a lot of construction supplies delivered to your home and then having the time and skills to quickly build a sound structure with those supplies.

THE MUSCULOSKELETAL SYSTEM

The musculoskeletal system includes your muscles, bones, tissues, and the foundational structure of your body, which helps you move and protects your internal organs. During pregnancy, you tend to gain at least 20 pounds from your baby, the placenta, extra blood volume, retained fluids, and increased fat storage, which results in around a 5 percent increase in lean muscle mass. Exercising can increase this lean muscle mass even more, improving your ability to meet the increased strain that pregnancy places on your body.

Hormonal and biomechanical shifts during pregnancy significantly affect the musculoskeletal system. As your baby grows and your belly expands, the increase in joint movement alters your balance and how you move your body. Additionally, as your weight increases (thanks to increased blood volume, your baby and all its accessories, and increased fat storage), there is more mechanical stress on this system.

These shifts in your body's stabilization and movement mechanics can lead to discomfort, including back and pelvic pain. Exercise can offset the side effects of these adaptations by increasing the muscular strength needed to counteract the change in balance, improve joint stability, and build the necessary strength to support the increased mass. Pain is not a requirement of pregnancy, and exercise is a simple (and nonmedical) solution.

Let's look at two specific adaptations that affect the musculoskeletal system: changes in hormones and changes in biomechanics, or how you move your body.

Hormonal Adaptations and Looser Joints

During pregnancy, your body secretes the hormone relaxin to loosen your muscles, joints, and ligaments to help your body stretch. This increases the mobility of your joints, particularly in the pelvis, to create more space for your baby during birth.

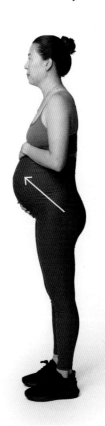

This enhanced joint mobility throughout your body can lead to pain, instability, and an elevated risk of injury.

Prenatal exercise, especially resistance training, can address these challenges by strengthening and coordinating supporting muscles, enhancing joint stability, and reinforcing ligaments and tendons for improved joint support, countering the effects of increased joint laxity during pregnancy. In turn, this reduces the likelihood of discomfort, strain, or injury.

Biomechanical Adaptations: Balance, Posture, and Movement

During pregnancy, your body undergoes biomechanical shifts, or adjustments in your balance, posture, and movement.

BALANCE: As your baby grows and your belly extends forward, your balance changes due to the shift in weight distribution. You may notice that you sway more forward and backward while standing, and you might adopt a wider stance to enhance stability and minimize side-to-side sway. Changes in your balance can increase the risk of falling. A study published in *Gait & Posture* suggests that around 25 percent of pregnant women experience falls due to diminished postural control.

Exercises that target the back, glutes, and hamstrings can help you counter this shift forward to maintain a more upright position and improve your balance. Chapters 4–6 will show you how to incorporate trimester specific exercises such as deadlifts, bent-over rows, cable pull-downs, and squats to offset this shift in your center of gravity.

POSTURE: During pregnancy, your usual postural habits become more pronounced. Before we discuss pregnancy-related changes, let's understand your existing habits that affect how you stand. As humans, we have normal asymmetry—our organs are not symmetrical, particularly our diaphragm, which is a key muscle involved in stabilization. Because of this, many of us tend to favor a right stance, where we put more weight on the right leg. This postural tendency means that our pelvis tends to be twisted toward the right, with the left hip forward and the right hip backward. This twist in the pelvis tends to result in the rib cage rotating more to the left. Another common posture favors external rotation in both hips (toes pointed outward), accompanied by a more pronounced arch in the back with the rib cage flaring upward.

Neither of these postures by themselves are problematic, but they can be if you cannot move out of them. During pregnancy, your positions tend to be more exaggerated, which can make it harder to transition to another position. When you're "stuck" in one position for too long, it can lead to muscle imbalances. Normally, muscles work together evenly, but imbalances mean one set of muscles is stronger or tighter than the other. This can cause misalignments and change how you move– which could contribute toward pelvic or low back pain and affect how you can open your pelvis during birth.

If you are "stuck" in these positions, you need to address the muscular balance with a combination of mobility and strengthening exercises. We discuss these specific exercises in chapter 5.

MOVEMENT: Pregnancy doesn't just affect how you balance and hold your body, but how you move your body as well. The biomechanical changes to your balance and posture also influence changes in the way you walk, also known as your *gait mechanics*. As pregnancy progresses, several changes occur in your gait cycle, which consists of the swing phase (when your foot is off the ground) and the stance phase (when your foot is on the ground).

These changes include moving at a slower pace, taking shorter steps, and spending less time with your feet off the ground. As a result, your steps become wider and your support base broadens. These adjustments happen gradually as your pregnancy advances. This change to your gait also affects how much your upper body and hips rotate as you move. The decreased rotation of your rib cage and pelvis can contribute to pelvic girdle pain and lower back discomfort.

The changes your body goes through during pregnancy are quite significant. They affect how you balance, your posture, and even the way you move. The good news is that exercising throughout your pregnancy can actually help you stay comfortable and pain-free as you prepare for birth. Part 2 will cover specific exercises to help you breeze through your pregnancy and postpartum period with greater ease.

REDUCING PRENATAL COMPLICATIONS

Prenatal exercise has been linked to reducing excessive maternal weight gain, potentially lowering the risk of prenatal complications, such as gestational hypertension (high blood pressure during pregnancy), preeclampsia, and gestational diabetes. According to research published in the *British Journal of Sports Medicine*, aerobic and resistance exercise several times a week has been shown to result in:

- 39 percent decreased risk of developing gestational hypertension
- 38 percent decreased risk of developing gestational diabetes
- 41 percent decreased risk of developing preeclampsia

If you develop a prenatal complication, your provider may recommend a medical induction of labor or even a Cesarean birth if your complication is severe. Reducing or delaying the onset of these complications can prolong your pregnancy and decrease the need for medical intervention at birth, which may improve your birth outcome.

PRENATAL COMPLICATIONS

PRENATAL COMPLICATION	WHAT IS IT?
Gestational Hypertension	Elevated blood pressure (>140/90) during pregnancy that develops after 20 weeks without impairing any major body organs
Preeclampsia	Elevated blood pressure during pregnancy that also impairs major body organs, such as the kidneys
Gestational Diabetes	Insulin resistance that develops during pregnancy due to the hormones of the placenta; can be diet controlled (type 1) or medication controlled (type 2)

WHEN NOT TO EXERCISE

FOR MOST PREGNANCIES CATEGORIZED as low risk, engaging in exercise is considered safe and offers a multitude of benefits that extend beyond pregnancy. Nonetheless, certain pre-existing conditions and prenatal complications might render exercise potentially harmful. To ensure the safety of both you and your baby, discuss your individual health circumstances with your health care provider.

When exercise can pose a risk:

- Severe respiratory or cardiovascular issues
- Placental abruption (the placenta separates from the uterine wall)
- Vasa previa (unprotected umbilical vessels)
- Uncontrolled type 1 diabetes
- Intrauterine growth restriction (IUGR)
- Active preterm labor
- Severe preeclampsia
- Cervical insufficiency (premature dilation of the cervix)

When exercising may not be advisable, but might be pursued under careful medical supervision:

- Vaginal bleeding
- Premature rupture of membranes
- Placenta previa (the placenta covers part of the cervix)
- Mild preeclampsia
- Mild respiratory or heart conditions
- Well-controlled type 1 diabetes
- Untreated thyroid disorder

In general, exercising throughout pregnancy is safe, but maintaining open communication with your provider is important, particularly if any limitations are warranted in your fitness routine due to existing or new medical conditions.

BENEFITS OF PRENATAL FITNESS FOR LABOR

Prenatal exercise not only supports a stronger and more comfortable pregnancy but can also prepare you for birth and improve your birth outcome. Prenatal exercise has been associated with:

- Shorter labor
- Decreased interventions
- Reduced likelihood of Cesarean birth
- Decreased use of forceps or vacuum for delivery

Exercising does not necessarily make you better at labor, but rather increases your stamina to maintain an upright position, change positions, and move for prolonged periods of time. This extra movement increases pressure on the cervix, which stimulates the release of prostaglandins that soften the cervix. In response, the pituitary gland releases oxytocin, causing the uterus to contract. This contraction increases pressure on the cervix and continues the feedback loop to speed up the labor process.

This increased stamina can also support pushing, as you may have to push for several hours. One reason that medical professionals use forceps or vacuum to help deliver a baby is because of maternal exhaustion. Due to increased endurance, you will likely be able to continue to push with sustained effort without the assistance of these interventions.

Additionally, shifting and changing positions helps your baby wiggle and rock through the pelvis more easily, decreasing the risk of a labor stall in which your baby gets "stuck." Preparation exercises can increase your ability to create more space in your pelvis for your baby, which can also reduce the risk of a labor stall. Labor stalls are one of the primary reasons for an unplanned Cesarean birth. It follows that if prenatal exercise can decrease the occurrence of a labor stall, then it can also decrease the likelihood of an unplanned C-section. We discuss labor stalls more in chapter 8.

Finally, regular prenatal exercise can reduce the occurrence, or delay the start, of some pregnancy complications. These problems may make a medical induction necessary, and depending on your provider, it could increase the risk of a C-section. In more serious cases, induction might not be possible, and an urgent C-section might be needed. We will discuss in chapter 2 how prenatal exercise can improve your baby's ability to handle the demands of labor. This extra resilience can reduce the likelihood of needing a C-section due to fetal distress during labor.

BENEFITS OF PRENATAL FITNESS FOR POSTPARTUM

Regular prenatal exercise can make it easier to recover from your birth. Establishing neuromuscular connections during pregnancy makes it easier to elicit these connections postpartum thanks to "muscle memory." You may feel very disconnected from your body after birth, a consequence of the rapid changes over nine months, suddenly reversed within hours or days due to hormonal shifts and substantial weight loss. However, the preestablished neuromuscular connections act as a repository of muscle memory, helping you reconnect with your body.

Additionally, prenatal fitness can reduce the potential for perinatal mood and anxiety disorders. Exercising throughout pregnancy not only reduces the risk and severity of postpartum depression but also lays the groundwork for continuing exercise into the postpartum period. Postpartum exercise has been correlated with a decreased risk of postpartum depression and other perinatal mood and anxiety disorders.

You may find that motivating yourself to work out during pregnancy is easier than in the postpartum. During pregnancy, your baby benefits from your workouts, and if it's your first baby, you don't have to worry about childcare. But in the postpartum, it may feel like the only one that benefits from your workouts is you, so it can be hard to prioritize yourself when there are so many other competing demands. However, the lack of exercise can affect your mental health!

Pelvic floor dysfunction or chronic pain (which can be improved with exercise) can also negatively affect your mental health. If it's hard for you to physically meet the demands of motherhood, such as picking up your baby or playing with them on the floor, it can affect your mental health. Plus, exercise boosts the concentration of mood-improving neurotransmitters like dopamine, which can improve sleep quality and cognitive function. So, taking time for yourself to exercise benefits not only you, but your entire family as well.

KEY TAKEAWAYS

Prenatal fitness significantly affects your pregnancy, birth, and postpartum journey. There are numerous physiological adaptations that occur during pregnancy that can be amplified with prenatal fitness, and these improvements have a significant effect on every system in your body. Prenatal exercise can increase your comfort throughout your entire pregnancy (remember, pain is not a requirement of pregnancy!). Prenatal exercise affects your birth outcome by decreasing the risk of prenatal complications and improving your movement capability to create space in your pelvis for your baby.

But the benefits of prenatal exercise are not limited to pregnancy and birth. Exercise can also positively affect your postpartum experience by improving your recovery after birth and laying the groundwork for a return to fitness to support your mental health as you enter motherhood.

In the next chapter, we will break down the benefits of prenatal fitness for your baby and how exercising can improve their in utero development, facilitate a smoother birth, and support their long-term health in infancy, childhood, and adulthood.

TWO
THE BENEFITS OF PRENATAL FITNESS FOR YOUR BABY

NOW THAT WE'VE DISCUSSED IN DETAIL how prenatal fitness can benefit you, let's talk about how it can benefit your growing baby. The majority of unsolicited advice regarding the safety of prenatal fitness tends to revolve around concerns about whether exercise can harm your baby. No mother would knowingly put her baby at risk, so when there's confusion about the safety of exercising during pregnancy, it may discourage you from exercising.

You may have been given cautious guidance on exercise, such as, "Don't lift more than 20 pounds." This is not based on any actual research or data. The "better safe than sorry" mentality that encourages you to decrease or avoid certain activities, "just in case," is harmful too, because decreasing physical activity during pregnancy can have negative effects on your baby's development. You may actually end up regretting it if you do not exercise.

While you can't inherit larger biceps from your parents, your physical activity during pregnancy can influence what your baby "inherits" in terms of their development. Prenatal exercise also helps with a smoother transition at birth and plays a role in your baby's long-term neuromuscular development during the early years of their life and beyond.

In this chapter, we'll explore the advantages of prenatal exercise for your baby and clarify why it is safe for your baby's well-being.

HOW PRENATAL EXERCISE BENEFITS YOUR BABY DURING PREGNANCY AND BIRTH

First, let's address common fears that you may have about exercising during pregnancy:

1. Will exercising affect my baby's growth and development in a negative way?
2. Will exercising cause me to go into preterm labor?

The answer to both of these questions is no. Exercising has not been shown to negatively affect your baby's growth and development. In fact, it can help better manage your baby's weight for better birth outcomes. Additionally, exercising has not been shown to cause preterm labor. There are other factors, such as physical stress and prenatal complications, that may cause preterm labor, but doing a daily workout is not one of them. Let's examine how exercise positively affects birth weight and labor more closely.

EXERCISE BENEFITS YOUR BABY'S BIRTH WEIGHT

Exercising throughout your pregnancy can improve your baby's birth outcome by better managing their birth weight. According to a study published in *Sports Medicine*, prenatal exercise has been associated with a decreased risk of a baby that is too large, known as *fetal macrosomia*, by 31 percent.

Risks of High Birth Weight

Birth weight is an important factor in neonatal health. A literature review published in the *International Journal of Environmental Research and Public Health* found that babies who are too large (or too small) at birth may have a higher rate of admission to the neonatal intensive care unit (NICU), have an increased risk of infection, and are more likely to have respiratory and metabolic issues.

A baby who is too large is also at greater risk for complications during birth. One such complication is known as *shoulder dystocia*, when the baby's shoulder gets caught in the pelvis after the head is born. This is considered a birth emergency and can result in lifelong complications or even death. Fortunately, shoulder dystocia is not a common occurrence and can be quickly resolved with a skilled provider and medical team.

According to research published in the *British Journal of Sports Medicine*, a too-large baby also increases the chance of an instrument-assisted delivery (using vacuum or forceps). Prenatal fitness can reduce the odds of instrument-assisted delivery by 24 percent. Although these tools can be helpful, they do come with certain risks, including potential harm to your baby's head and neck and an increased risk of damage to your perineal area and pelvic floor. In addition to the baby's size, another common reason for instrument-assisted delivery is maternal fatigue: The mother is too tired to push effectively. Both of these risk factors can be mitigated by exercising and improving your endurance during pregnancy.

Finally, if your provider suspects that your baby is too big, they may recommend scheduling a C-section, as your baby may have difficulty fitting through your pelvis. Even though your baby can shape-shift as they move through the pelvis and larger babies can be born vaginally, a larger baby may take a longer time to descend through the pelvis (which can be an issue depending on your provider's patience).

Risks of Low Birth Weight

On the other end of the spectrum is the concern that prenatal exercise will negatively affect your baby's growth, causing them to be too small. This is a problem because a baby that is too small is at greater risk for premature birth, medical induction of labor, and Cesarean birth. Once born, a low-birth-weight baby also has difficulty regulating body temperature, breathing, and feeding.

There are two main fears that may contribute to the incorrect notion that prenatal exercise is associated with low-birth-weight babies. The first concern is that exercising affects blood flow to the baby, and this decreased oxygen availability could affect their growth. The second concern is that exercise can negatively affect your placenta's growth or potentially detach it from the uterine wall. Let's discuss why these two concerns are false—and in fact the opposite is true, thanks to prenatal exercise.

The first misconception that exercise during pregnancy diverts blood flow from the uterus to the muscles, reducing oxygen for the baby and hindering growth, has been debunked. If your baby's oxygen availability is decreased, it will increase their heart rate. Fluctuations in a baby's heart rate that are within normal limits do not indicate a problem. In fact, low- to moderate-intensity prenatal exercise shows no or minimal effect on the blood flow between the uterus and the placenta. Additionally, levels of the hormone erythropoietin, which increases red blood cells when oxygen levels are low, have been shown to be lower in babies born to mothers who exercised during pregnancy.

The second misconception, that exercise will affect your placenta in a negative way, such as causing it to detach from the uterine wall, is also not true. The placenta provides your baby with oxygen and nutrients, removes metabolic waste, produces hormones that help your baby grow, and can even pass immunity to your baby. The placenta is very well protected in the uterus, and prenatal exercise does not increase any risk to your placenta's function or attachment. In fact, prenatal exercise can improve your placenta's function by increasing its volume and growth rate; if your placenta is larger, its functional capacity may increase. Weight-bearing activities, such as lifting weights, may positively affect placental growth more so than nonweight-bearing activities, such as aerobic activity.

Finally, according to research published in the *British Journal of Sports Medicine*, prenatal exercise can reduce your risk of developing gestational hypertension or blood pressure issues, two factors in low birth weight, by up to 39 percent and will therefore improve your baby's development in utero.

EXERCISE BENEFITS YOUR BABY DURING LABOR AND DELIVERY

We have discussed how the management of your baby's weight can improve birth outcomes for both of you, but let's dive deeper into how your baby will better tolerate the stress of labor thanks to your exercising throughout your pregnancy.

Regular exercise during pregnancy benefits the baby by increasing their blood volume, which ensures better oxygen and nutrient transportation during labor and helps them cope with labor stress. When uterine contractions temporarily restrict the baby's blood supply, their oxygen reserve helps maintain their oxygen levels.

One way we know that babies of mothers who exercise throughout their pregnancy better tolerate the stresses of labor is because they have lower levels of the hormone erythropoietin (produced in response to low oxygen levels) and a reduced occurrence of meconium, or stool in the amniotic fluid, which can be a sign of fetal distress. These two factors suggest that these babies are more resilient during labor compared to those whose mothers didn't exercise.

Another fear is that exercise will cause preterm labor, or cause your water to break spontaneously. We'll discuss this in more depth in chapter 3 on pages 33 and 35, but in a nutshell, the data show that there is no association between prenatal exercise and preterm labor. Rather, thanks to your workouts throughout your pregnancy, your baby will reap the benefits of improved cardiovascular reserve and resiliency. And this continues into the postpartum period, as you'll soon see!

HOW PRENATAL EXERCISE BENEFITS YOUR BABY IN THE POSTPARTUM

It should come as no surprise that prenatal exercise also enhances your baby's experience after birth—and the benefits go beyond just the first few days or weeks postpartum. In fact, your workouts can affect their lifelong health!

The first assessment to check your baby's well-being after birth is their APGAR score. This score rates a baby's appearance, pulse, grimace, activity, and respiration. Each category can receive a score of 0 to 2, and the total score can range from 0 to 10. A higher score indicates a smoother transition to life outside the womb, while a lower score may signal that the baby requires more attention and support during this time. Babies of mothers who exercised during pregnancy typically have higher APGAR scores compared with babies of nonexercising mothers.

According to a study in the *British Journal of Sports Medicine*, this smoother transition from womb to world also includes your baby regaining their birth weight more rapidly, exhibiting stable blood glucose levels, and maintaining their body temperature even with less body fat. Thus, the benefits of prenatal fitness are evident in the days after birth.

Prenatal exercise can positively affect your baby's brain and nervous system development in utero. Research published in *Medicine & Science in Sports & Exercise* and *Journal of Physical Activity and Health* has shown that these babies have improved neuromotor development with improved language and cognitive development both as newborns and as children. So, your workouts during your pregnancy can positively affect your baby not only in utero and at birth, but well into their elementary school years and beyond.

Furthermore, if you are dedicated to exercising during your pregnancy, it's realistic that you'll stick to an exercise routine after giving birth. Modeling an active lifestyle for your children can motivate them to prioritize fitness as they grow older. The advantages of prenatal fitness for children can have long-lasting effects into adulthood because it encourages them to participate in physical activities that enhance general motor skills and specific sports skills, which in turn motivates them to maintain an active lifestyle throughout their childhood and adult lives.

KEY TAKEAWAYS

One of the primary concerns regarding prenatal exercise is whether it might have a detrimental effect on your baby's growth and development, potentially affecting their well-being both before and after birth. However, there is no evidence that suggests any negative effects of exercising during pregnancy on your baby. In fact, research consistently highlights the substantial benefits of prenatal exercise.

Studies have repeatedly shown that exercising during pregnancy can actually enhance your baby's in utero development. It contributes to the growth of their brain and nervous system, improves their ability to respond to stress, and facilitates a smoother transition after birth. As infants and children, those who were exposed to prenatal exercise tend to exhibit enhanced neuromotor function, improved language skills, and better cognitive development.

You can have confidence that maintaining an exercise routine throughout your pregnancy is not only safe but also incredibly advantageous for your baby. Choosing not to exercise solely to err on the side of caution can potentially have a negative effect on your baby's health, not only during your pregnancy and birth, but also throughout their childhood and into their adult years.

PART 2

PRENATAL FITNESS

NOW THAT YOU UNDERSTAND THE BENEFITS of prenatal fitness for you and your baby, it's time to start exploring how to incorporate prenatal fitness into your daily routine with considerations for each trimester. In this section, you will learn how to confidently approach exercise safely throughout your pregnancy, as I debunk common myths associated with prenatal fitness.

You'll learn that *what* you do to exercise throughout your pregnancy is not as important as *how* you exercise throughout your pregnancy. In this part of the book, I will share how to approach your workouts with positioning and breathing to minimize injuries and optimize your performance. Then you will learn several beneficial exercises, plus modifications for each trimester, to incorporate into your prenatal workout. These exercises will keep you strong and comfortable throughout your pregnancy as you prepare for birth, whether it be a vaginal birth or a Cesarean.

In this section, I also share solutions for common issues experienced in each trimester, such as low back pain, pelvic girdle pain, and sleeping issues. Pain is not a requirement of pregnancy—and you will fully recognize that there is a lot you can do to find pain relief.

THREE
APPROACHING PRENATAL FITNESS

AS I DISCUSSED IN CHAPTERS 1 AND 2, exercising is incredibly beneficial for you and your baby throughout pregnancy, while not exercising may be associated with greater risks. This chapter explains how to approach prenatal fitness, how to design a prenatal fitness routine, and how to select the best exercises for your prenatal workouts. The goal of this chapter is to teach you how to use prenatal fitness to support your pregnancy and your preparation for birth, regardless of whether you are planning a vaginal or Cesarean birth.

During my first pregnancy, I had no clue what I should have done to maintain a level of fitness for myself and my baby. I thought I could just continue doing my prepregnancy workouts and just skip any of the exercises I had heard were "unsafe." For my subsequent pregnancies, I followed the prenatal fitness programs I developed for MamasteFit. The differences in my prenatal comfort, labor experiences, and postpartum recoveries were drastic, solidifying the importance of an intentional and well-informed program. More than likely, you, too, have found yourself inundated with conflicting information and unsolicited advice about how to exercise safely during pregnancy. Therefore, this chapter will start by debunking some of the widespread misconceptions about prenatal fitness.

DEBUNKING PRENATAL FITNESS MYTHS

These days, social media often showcases polarizing reactions to pregnant athletes exercising. Ranging from uplifting admiration to unsettling negativity, these comments can create an environment where working out during pregnancy feels anything but safe. I will debunk common misunderstandings surrounding prenatal fitness so you can feel confident in the safety and advantages of exercising, benefiting both you and your baby.

MYTH I: EXERCISING DURING PREGNANCY INCREASES YOUR RISK OF MISCARRIAGE AND PRETERM LABOR.

This myth is false. Exercising during your pregnancy, including lifting heavy weights, does not increase your risk of miscarriage, nor does it increase your risk of preterm labor (labor before 37 weeks). The fear of miscarriage can be a huge deterrence to exercising throughout your pregnancy, especially if you have numerous people giving you unsolicited advice about your fitness routine and suggesting it is putting your baby in harm's way.

In multiple randomized controlled trials published in the *British Journal of Sports Medicine* and the *Journal of Clinical Medicine*, researchers found no significant associations between exercising during pregnancy and the occurrence of miscarriage. In these studies, exercises included low- to moderate-intensity aerobic exercise and resistance training, with workout durations of 20 to 65 minutes per session. A Norwegian study published in the *BMJ Open Sport & Exercise Medicine* also found that exercising more than 150 minutes per week, the minimum recommendation for pregnancy, did not increase the risk of miscarriage.

The majority of miscarriages are due to chromosomal abnormalities, or a fetus that is, sadly, not compatible with life. In other words, there is nothing that you could have done to cause it, and unfortunately, nothing anyone could have done to prevent the pregnancy loss. Miscarriage does happen in one out of every four pregnancies, so it is tragically more common than many of us realize.

Furthermore, exercising during pregnancy does not correlate with a higher likelihood of preterm labor. This myth that exercise can cause preterm labor may originate from the recommendation of bed rest, which is often prescribed to prolong pregnancies at risk of delivery before 37 weeks. Bed rest may be prescribed if you are carrying twins or multiples, are experiencing preterm labor, have a short cervix, or are at risk of early water breaking.

Nevertheless, recent studies in the *Canadian Medical Association Open Access Journal* and *Australian and Current Opinion in Obstetrics and Gynecology* have indicated that bed rest does not effectively prolong pregnancies when complications risking early delivery arise. Research reviews in the *Canadian Medical Association Open Access Journal* have found that one week of bed rest can actually worsen newborn outcomes. Additionally, bed rest could result in muscular atrophy from lack of physical activity, contributing to discomfort and pain. Current research in the *Australian and New Zealand Journal of Obstetrics and Gynecology* agrees that bed rest is an outdated practice.

The misconception that exercise might lead to miscarriage or preterm labor, along with negative commentary questioning the safety of staying active, can intensify the burden of responsibility you bear if unfortunate events occur. Instead of offering empathy in moments of grief and loss, these notions place undue blame on the woman.

MYTH 2: YOU NEED TO BE REALLY CAUTIOUS ABOUT RAISING YOUR CORE BODY TEMPERATURE WITH EXERCISE.

It is important to exercise in appropriate environments and maintain proper hydration, but you do not need to be overly fearful of overheating in a temperature-controlled environment.

While it's true that if your core body temperature does increase, it could have detrimental effects on the baby, the good news is your body is much better adapted to keeping you cool during pregnancy. This is due to the increase in blood volume and the physiological adaptations of the cardiovascular system. According to research published in *Exercising Through Your Pregnancy*, tolerance to heat stress increases by 30 percent in the early part of pregnancy and at least 70 percent in the third trimester. Increased blood volume increases your skin blood flow, which enhances your ability to keep yourself cool and maintain your core body temperature. Even exercising at a 65 percent effort level in late pregnancy does not increase your core body temperature. So, the concern that your workouts can cause harm to your baby due to overheating is not as much of a concern as you may have been led to believe.

Still, it is recommended to avoid prolonged intense exercise in extremely hot and humid environments, and to maintain proper hydration during workouts.

MYTH 3: WEIGHTLIFTING WILL CAUSE A TIGHT PELVIC FLOOR AND MAKE LABOR HARDER.

This myth is promoted by some outdated medical providers and birth professionals; however, the truth is more nuanced and complex than many realize.

It's important to clarify that merely participating in weightlifting does not inherently result in pelvic floor tightness that disrupts labor. Rather, *how* you lift weights and move your body can correlate with muscular tension patterns in your body.

Much like our discussion in chapter 1 concerning shifts in biomechanics due to postural and movement tendencies, performing repetitive motions and neglecting other movement directions can affect muscle tension.

For instance, if your weightlifting routine primarily encompasses movements within the sagittal plane (forward and backward)—such as exercises like clean and jerks or squats that emphasize hip extension and external rotation—while neglecting movements favoring internal rotation at the hip and rounding of the back, you might indeed experience heightened tension in the pelvic floor. This tension could negatively affect your prenatal comfort and potentially hinder the birthing process.

To counteract this potential adverse effect, it's important to incorporate exercises across all three planes of motion: forward and backward (sagittal plane), side to side (frontal plane), and rotation (transverse plane). This approach requires various spinal and hip orientations, activating different muscles during a workout.

Here are examples of strength exercises in the three planes of motion:

- **Lower Body:**
  » Squats (sagittal plane)
  » Lateral band walk (frontal plane)
  » Split squat with hip internal and external rotation (transverse plane)

- **Upper Body:**
  » Bench press (sagittal plane)
  » Lat pull-down (frontal plane)
  » Pallof press and rotation (transverse plane)

The act of weightlifting alone does not inherently lead to a tense pelvic floor and issues in your birth. But repeatedly moving in a singular plane of motion while neglecting the other planes can affect your ability to create space in your pelvis for birth. So, it is important to be intentional about the types of exercises you are including in your prenatal workout routine and ensure that there is a diverse array of exercises. This book will help you do just that.

MYTH 4: YOU SHOULD NEVER RUN OR JUMP DURING PREGNANCY.

The truth behind this myth is, "It depends." This myth might originate from worries that high-impact activities could lead to your water breaking spontaneously before you reach 37 weeks. Nevertheless, research published in the *British Journal of Sports Medicine* has demonstrated that this is not the case. Risk factors for preterm premature rupture of membranes (PPROM) involve various prenatal complications that are unrelated to prenatal exercise or high-impact activities.

High-impact activities, such as running and jumping, will likely not be comfortable throughout the entire duration of your pregnancy. As your pregnancy progresses, the load on your pelvic floor, joints, and musculoskeletal system also increases and can be easily overwhelmed by high-impact exercise.

If you are running or jumping and you feel comfortable and pain-free, it is likely fine to continue doing those higher-impact activities. Some people can continue running or jumping until giving birth without complications.

However, it's crucial to watch out for signs that higher-impact exercises may no longer be suitable. These signs can include sensations of pelvic floor heaviness, incontinence, lower abdominal or back pain, and general discomfort or pain during high-impact activities. If any of these symptoms arise, it may be better to shift to lower-impact activities like swimming, using a stationary bike, or walking. If modification is necessary, remember that it's only a temporary adjustment. You can eventually return to these activities after recovering postpartum.

MYTH 5: YOU SHOULD *NEVER* TWIST OR USE CLOSED HIP POSITIONS DURING YOUR WORKOUTS.

Some birth professionals have raised concerns that twisting during pregnancy could potentially result in placental complications or harm to the baby. However, these concerns lack a solid foundation in research and evidence. This myth is false. While engaging in deep abdominal compressions and intense twisting might not be advisable during pregnancy, it's important to note that controlled twisting and rotation of the spine and hips are actually essential throughout this period.

Maintaining proper spine and hip rotation throughout pregnancy is essential for overall well-being. Failing to incorporate rotation into your movements can lead to various issues, such as lower back pain, pelvic pain, and even the potential for labor to stall. When you neglect rotation, the burden on the lower back intensifies because it compensates for the lack of movement in the hips and upper back, resulting in pain and discomfort. Additionally, the inability to rotate the hips adversely affects pelvic positioning, potentially reducing space within the pelvis. Rotation is crucial for prenatal comfort and birth preparation, and dismissing twists and rotation exacerbates these challenges.

Another misconception is that twisting during pregnancy should only include open twists. Open twists are twists in which the hips maintain an open position or externally rotate, moving away from the midline—the belly is "open" to space. There is a strong objection to closed hip positions, characterized by internal rotation at the hip where the belly pushes into the thigh. However, it's important to note that solely focusing on external hip rotation can potentially have unintended consequences for prenatal comfort and for labor. The inability to access internal hip rotation has been associated with posterior pelvic floor restriction, pelvic pain, and labor stalls due to limited space in the lower pelvis.

In summary, you should absolutely twist and rotate during pregnancy. The misconception that twisting is dangerous is incorrect, and the lack of rotation could cause more complications during your pregnancy and labor. In the following trimester-specific chapters, you'll find several rotational exercises that can improve mobility and decrease pain throughout your pregnancy.

MYTH 6: NEVER EXERCISE ON YOUR BACK.

Another common recommendation is to never exercise on your back or in a supine (lying down) position. This recommendation is based on the idea that if you are supine, the vena cava, or the large artery behind the uterus, can be compressed, and it can decrease uterine blood flow and be harmful to your baby.

Research published in the *American Journal of Perinatology* and the *British Journal of Sports Medicine* demonstrates that typically before 28 weeks, exercising in a supine position for 2 to 5 minutes at a time should not cause complications. Generally, after 28 weeks, you can continue to exercise in a supine position for 2 to 5 minutes if there are no side effects, such as dizziness or lightheadedness. If you do begin to experience side effects from being in a supine position, roll to the left side to rest until your symptoms subside.

If you continue to experience symptoms in a supine position, modify your supine exercises to an upright or inclined variation, such as modifying the bench press to the standing chest or incline dumbbell press. In each trimester-specific chapter, you can find more modifications for supine exercises.

MYTH 7: IF YOU DID A WORKOUT ROUTINE BEFORE PREGNANCY, YOU COULD CONTINUE IT DURING PREGNANCY.

The common recommendation for prenatal fitness is that you can do what you did before pregnancy, making slight adjustments such as reducing weights or lowering intensity. While this guidance contains elements of truth, it overlooks several crucial aspects.

First, this myth suggests that those who were inactive before pregnancy must refrain from exercising or initiating a new routine, which is not true. It is safe to start a brand-new workout routine during pregnancy, even if you have never done that exercise before. However, it's important not to approach this new routine like you've been engaged in it for years. Start gently, gradually progressing to prevent excessive soreness.

Second, if you were active before pregnancy, the assumption that you can essentially replicate your former workout with minor adjustments is not entirely accurate. While it is generally safe to continue to do most of the exercises that you did before pregnancy, you'll likely need to modify some exercises for comfort and you may need to omit certain exercises altogether. For example, squatting with a barbell is often viable throughout pregnancy, but if you feel discomfort in the lower back during the squat's descent, you may want to switch to a box squat for added support. Again, each trimester-specific chapter provides modifications for various exercises.

In general, it's possible to continue familiar exercises from before pregnancy, but you'll need to make adaptations. Additionally, starting a new workout routine while pregnant is absolutely doable, as long as you gradually ease into it. This is discussed more in chapter 5.

FOUNDATIONAL PRINCIPLES OF PRENATAL FITNESS

Your prenatal fitness journey starts with the right mindset. It's important to approach pregnancy with an open mind because your expectations may be different from your reality. Pregnancy brings a range of sensations and symptoms that can fluctuate each day, such as varying energy levels, nausea, or heartburn. The right mindset can help guide you toward the exercises and intensity levels that best support your pregnancy in each trimester.

There is a huge piece of prenatal fitness that involves the act of letting go. This can be challenging to do if you associate your sport as a part of your identity—it may feel like pieces of you are slowly being taken away as your pregnancy progresses. I've worked with many athletes who are desperately trying to maintain a workout routine that is similar to their prepregnancy practice because it feels like the last hold they have on their premotherhood identity. Additionally, if you are an athlete, you may be used to pushing through discomfort. It is important not to ignore signs from your body. Honoring how your body feels each day and adjusting your workouts to accommodate those needs will support a better pregnancy experience and prepare you mentally for birth—and for motherhood.

Be flexible with your workout approach. This includes shortening the workout if you are tired or increasing the intensity if energized. You may need to modify exercises or omit specific movements. You might change your workout entirely, like going for an easy walk instead of weightlifting. As you embrace the concept of mental flexibility in your prenatal fitness approach, you're not just adapting your workouts—you're also welcoming a mindful approach to pregnancy and birth preparation that extends into the postpartum period.

After you've established your mindset and approach to prenatal fitness, the next step is to focus on how you do the exercises. How you perform the exercises is more important than which exercises you choose to do. The key things to consider are:

- **Core stabilization:** How well your torso can maintain its position during movement
- **Position and alignment:** How your joints are set up to stabilize your body during movement
- **Pressure management:** How your breathing affects your stabilization
- **Breath-to-movement coordination:** How you combine your movements and your breathing to enhance your stabilization and performance

Let's look at each in turn.

CORE STABILIZATION

The first foundational principle of functional movement is core stabilization, or the ability to maintain your torso position as your arms and legs move. This includes your static positioning (when you're standing still) and your more dynamic and functional movement (when you're lifting weights or running). All of your movements originate from the core canister.

The core canister comprises the respiratory diaphragm, transverse abdominis and internal oblique muscles, multifidus, and pelvic floor. These deep core muscles work together to maintain stability. Your muscles can respond to demand best in a midrange position, allowing them to adapt to different demands quickly. A neutral spine is considered the ideal midrange position for your core. This means that when your spine is in a neutral position, it sets up your core to best stabilize and manage pressure. This can improve your athletic performance but more importantly reduces core and pelvic floor issues. Chapter 4 explores core exercises that you can do throughout your pregnancy.

POSITION AND ALIGNMENT

The second foundational principle is getting your joints in the right position. When your joints are properly aligned, your muscles can work better. Some joints need to be stable and rigid, like your lower back (lumbar spine) and knees, while other joints need to be more mobile, like your upper back (thoracic spine), hips, and ankles. Generally, you want to lift weights in a neutral spine position, as it sets your joints up to best stabilize without excessive strain and sets your muscles up best to function.

Certain exercises benefit from maintaining a stable and rigid neutral spine position. For instance, excessive lumbar spine movement could increase your risk of lower back injury in movements like back squats or deadlifts. In other exercises, it's important that the hips and spine have the ability to rotate, such as lunges, where internal and external rotation at the hip is vital for pelvic stability. In both cases, aiming for a neutral spine position is preferred instead of arching or rounding your back.

Still, there isn't one perfect posture or position that you should always be in. Even the commonly recommended "perfect posture" of neutral can cause problems if held for prolonged periods. In the fitness world, there's a saying that your

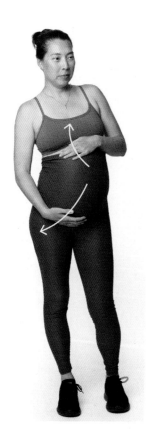

best posture is your next one. Being able to easily change positions with control is more important than sticking to one rigid posture. So, being able to find a neutral spine position, in addition to arching or rounding in the back, plus being able to rotate and laterally move the spine, is crucial for stabilization and an important aspect of fitness. (However, you may need to reserve the more mobile movements of your spine for lighter weights or bodyweight movements, as opposed to squats and deadlifts.)

If you get "stuck" in one posture or position for too long, it can lead to problematic muscle imbalances. Normally, muscles work together evenly, but an imbalance means one set of muscles is stronger or tighter than the other. For example, if you tend to favor a right stance posture (like the figure on the left), some muscles become overly tight, while others lengthen too much and cannot counterbalance the uneven pull. This results in your pelvis rotating in different directions: the left side moves forward while the right side moves backward.

On the left side:

- The hip flexor, quad, and glutes shorten to pull the pelvis forward.
- The inner thigh and hamstring are lengthened and usually weaker.

On the right side:

- The hamstring and adductor shorten to pull the pelvis backward.
- The quad and glutes are lengthened and usually weaker.

The postural tendency to favor a right stance is not usually a problem, because we have natural asymmetry. But it can become an issue when you get "stuck" there or have difficulty transitioning from that stance to another. The resulting muscular imbalances can cause misalignments and change how you move, which could contribute to pelvic or lower back pain.

Your postural habits also affect how your pelvic floor functions. When you tend to arch your back (like the figure on the right), it tightens the back part of your pelvic floor, while stretching the front part excessively. This imbalance may make it harder for you to release muscle tension and may cause problems with incontinence.

It's important to be able to stabilize your core to alleviate lower back and pelvic pain, and you'll need to be able to release tightened muscles to allow your baby to easily pass through the birth canal.

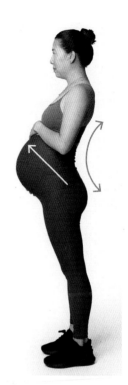

MUSCLE LOCATION AND FUNCTION QUICK REFERENCE CHART

MUSCLE	LOCATION	FUNCTION
Adductor	Inner thigh	Bring the legs together Rotates the hip internally
Hamstring	Back thigh	Pulls the pelvis backward Rotates the hip internally
Glute (Butt Muscle)	Back of hip	Straightens the hip Rotates the hip externally Separates the legs
Quadricep (Quad)	Front of thigh	Bends the hip Straightens the knee
Hip Flexor	Front of hip	Bends the hip
Pelvic Floor	Base of pelvis	Supports pelvic organs Providers sphincter control Stabilizes the spine

ANATOMICAL TERM QUICK REFERENCE CHART

BIOMECHANICAL CHANGE	DESCRIPTION
External Rotation of the Hip	Toes point outward Open hip position
Internal Rotation of the Hip	Toes point inward Closed hip position
Abduction	Legs move apart
Adduction	Legs move together
Anterior Pelvic Tilt	Pelvis rotates forward More arch in lower back
Posterior Pelvic Tilt	Pelvis rotates backward Butt tucks under Flatter appearance of the lower back
Rib Cage Flare or Spinal Extension	Arching in the back as the front side of the rib cage elevates upward

If you find yourself getting "stuck" in certain postures or positions, you need to address the muscular imbalance with a combination of mobility and strengthening exercises. We discuss these specific exercises in chapter 5 starting on page 76.

PRESSURE MANAGEMENT

The third foundational principle is the ability to manage pressure. This means using your breath to change the internal pressure in the thoracic and abdominal cavity based on demand. Increased pressure stabilizes the spine. In contrast, increased muscular activation can counter increased pressure to protect the points of least resistance, such as your pelvic floor or abdominal separation.

But pressure management does not mean increasing pressure as high as possible and increasing muscular activation as much as possible with every breath. You need to adjust the pressure based on the stabilization demand. When more stability is needed, such as when lifting heavy weights, increased intra-abdominal pressure

(IAP) provides support. Conversely, IAP can also be lower when stability demands are lower, like when sitting. It is essential to adjust IAP according to the demand rather than always using maximum or insufficient effort.

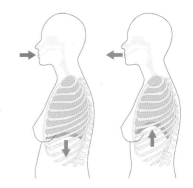

However, during pregnancy, you don't want to generate incredibly high levels of IAP, as the abdominal wall and pelvic floor are less able to withstand high levels of pressure. Therefore, you'll want to decrease the overall demand during lifts and reduce your effort level according to the stage of your pregnancy. We'll discuss this more in the trimester-specific chapters.

So, how do you manage pressure? With your breathing. Diaphragmatic breathing uses the diaphragm to adjust the pressure within your thoracic and abdominal cavities. Your breathing cycle involves two components: inhalation and exhalation.

Inhalation

When you inhale, your diaphragm moves down, flattens, and increases pressure in the abdominal cavity. This causes the abdominal wall, back musculature, and pelvic floor to expand outward and lengthen. This increased pressure stabilizes the spine and can be observed when someone lifts heavy weights; inhaling to expand their torso increases core stabilization before starting the lift.

Lengthening (eccentric) movements involves two key points:

- **First,** we're typically stronger during the lengthening phase of an exercise. Lowering a weight with gravity is often easier than lifting it against gravity. This strength advantage in the eccentric phase means that during the breathing cycle, inhaling (eccentric) provides more stability than exhaling (concentric).

- **Second,** the eccentric part of a movement gathers energy to produce power. This is similar to stretching a rubber band: When released, the band recoils and propels forward. This happens because the band accumulates energy as it's stretched, using that stored energy to spring into action. Similarly, when you inhale, the lengthening part of your breath accumulates energy, enhancing your athletic performance.

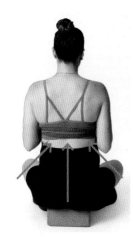

Exhalation

When you exhale, the core canister returns to its original resting position or contracts to increase muscular force to counter the increased pressure from external demands, such as lifting weights.

Exhalations are the shortening (concentric) portion of our breathing cycle, and there are two ways you can exhale. In the first, you activate your muscles to counter the increase in pressure. This option is best if you are lifting something heavy, where you may want to exhale against exertion to counter the increased IAP. But remember, the concentric portion of our movements are not as strong as the eccentric portion, so exhaling to flex your abs is not an efficient stabilization strategy. With the second option, you exhale to release or relax, so the core canister returns to its resting position. This exhalation strategy is best when you are at rest or doing a low-stabilization-demand task, such as sitting or walking.

BREATH-TO-MOVEMENT COORDINATION

Now that you understand breathing mechanics, the last foundational principle is coordinating your breath and movement to improve stabilization. If you enhance stabilization at key points during your lifts, you can improve your performance and minimize pressure-management-related issues, such as incontinence, pelvic organ prolapse, or hernias.

How do you remember whether to inhale or exhale with an exercise? Inhales are the eccentric, or lengthening, portion of your breath cycle, while exhales are the concentric, or shortening, portion of your breath cycle. You can then match that portion of your breath cycle to the portion of the exercise you are in. When you are moving with gravity, such as when lowering in a squat, you are in the lengthening (eccentric) portion of the lift. You want to inhale to increase pressure before lowering, or during

QUICK REFERENCE CHART FOR
BREATH-TO-MOVEMENT COORDINATION

Inhalation	Moving *with* gravity Eccentric portion of the exercise Feeling more stretch in this part of the exercise
Exhalation	Moving *against* gravity Concentric portion of the exercise Typically, the harder part of the exercise

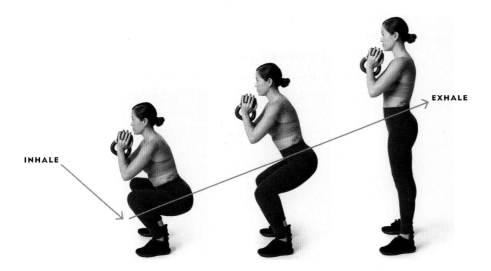

INHALE

EXHALE

your descent. When moving against gravity, such as when standing up from the bottom of a squat, you are in the shortening (concentric) portion of the lift. You want to exhale to increase muscular activation and counter the increased IAP.

When it comes to breath-to-movement coordination, there are three breathing strategies to consider. In general, you inhale when moving *with* gravity and exhale when moving *against* gravity (strategy 1). But there are other options, depending on your circumstances. If you are in your third trimester and lifting lighter weights, then you may want to use a less-advanced breathing strategy (strategy 2). On the other hand, depending on your fitness level and the demand of your lift, you may want to use a more advanced breathing technique (strategy 3). Let's look at each strategy in turn.

Breathing Strategy 1: Inhale when moving *with* gravity. Exhale when moving *against* gravity.

The first breathing strategy has moderate levels of IAP and is the most commonly used throughout pregnancy. In this breathing strategy, you inhale as you lower in a movement or move *with* gravity. Then, you will exhale as you stand up or move *against* gravity. For example, you inhale as you lower in a squat, then exhale as you stand up for the entire duration of the movement. This is a synchronized effort, where you are moving and breathing at the same time.

Breathing Strategy 2: Inhale when moving *with* gravity. Begin to exhale, *then* move against gravity.

The second breathing strategy creates the least IAP, which will be most manageable in the third trimester, early postpartum, or at times when there is lower stabilization demand. This breathing strategy can be great for bodyweight movements as

POOR BREATHING STRATEGIES

Because breathing is how you manage pressure, improper breathing strategies can increase pelvic floor dysfunction, worsen abdominal separation, and affect your performance during your workouts. The following poor (but common) breathing strategies should be avoided during your prenatal workouts.

Reverse Breathing

Reverse breathing is the opposite of diaphragmatic breathing. In reverse breathing, when you inhale, you lift the shoulders and chest to inhale upward, then exhale to push down. This breathing strategy increases pressure downward onto the pelvic floor, also known as *bearing down*. Bearing down may feel like a downward sensation in the pelvic floor, similar to if you are having a bowel movement or a feeling of pelvic floor heaviness. Excessive bearing down on the pelvic floor can worsen pelvic floor–related issues, such as pelvic organ prolapse, increased pelvic floor tension, constipation, or incontinence. This breathing strategy also does not help manage pressure properly and can hinder your performance in your lifts.

Belly Breathing

Belly breathing emphasizes belly expansion during inhalation, as opposed to rib cage expansion. This breathing technique tends to be popular in yoga settings and may be used as a way to coach diaphragmatic breathing because it is easier to witness the belly expanding with inhalations and pulling in with exhalations.

Although this breathing strategy is moving the diaphragm in the correct direction, it emphasizes the expansion of the weakened abdominal wall as opposed to the expansion of the more robust back musculature. You do want some expansion in the belly as you inhale, but this breathing strategy focuses all of the pressure from your inhalation into the belly. Overemphasis on belly expansion can worsen abdominal separation and is not an optimal stabilization strategy for exercise, as it does not increase the rigidity of the spine.

Gripping or Clenching

If you are gripping your abs or clenching your pelvic floor muscles while breathing, you are redirecting pressure in a suboptimal way. When you grip your abs, it can increase pressure on the pelvic floor muscles during inhalation because the abdominal wall is not expanding at all. When you clench the pelvic floor muscles while breathing, it can increase pressure on the abdominal wall. Both breathing strategies alter the stabilization strategy of the deep core musculature—essentially, one gear of the system is stuck, affecting how the other muscles of this coordinated system work.

well, because the demand is lower and does not require high levels of IAP. In this strategy, you inhale as you lower in a movement or move *with* gravity. Then, you start to exhale before you begin the ascent, or move *against* gravity, to prepare the pelvic floor and core, and continue to exhale as you finish the exercise. This strategy can help you learn each step of the breathing cycle and coordinate it with your movement as you focus on one portion at a time (exhale, then lift).

Breathing Strategy 3: Inhale, *then* move with gravity.
Exhale when moving *against* gravity.

The final breathing strategy, and the most advanced of the breathing strategies, is to hold your breath during the eccentric portions of movement and then exhale at some point during your ascent or movement against gravity. You can exhale at any point during the concentric phase, but typically you exhale near the end of the lift. For example, you inhale to increase IAP, then lower in your squat. Then, you begin to stand up and exhale at some point during the ascent, typically in the last quarter of the ascent. This breathing strategy can be used throughout pregnancy, but the amount of IAP generated is lower than prepregnancy.

How can you determine which is the best breathing strategy to use for your workout? If you are able to maintain optimal form and you do not feel increased pressure on the pelvic floor during the concentric portion of the exercise, the breathing strategy is appropriate for you. If you feel increased heaviness on the pelvic floor, then you should choose an easier breathing strategy and lower the intensity of the exercise.

DESIGNING YOUR IDEAL PRENATAL FITNESS ROUTINE

Now that we've debunked some myths and discussed our core principles, let's get into the nitty-gritty of actually designing your prenatal fitness routine.

WORKOUT DURATION

When developing a prenatal fitness routine, first ensure that you are exceeding the minimum workout duration requirements (*at least* 150 minutes of moderate-intensity activity per week). You can split the 150 minutes (or more) across several days. Choosing the exercise that you find most enjoyable is a good start, but it can be helpful to incorporate resistance training in addition to walking, yoga, or other light-impact exercises you enjoy. We will break down exercise recommendations per trimester in the upcoming chapters. For now, here is a sample 5-day workout routine, in which you can do 30 minutes or more per day to meet the minimum recommendation.

SAMPLE DAY ROUTINE

DAY 1	DAY 2	DAY 3	DAY 4	DAY 5
Lower-body resistance training with mobility	Upper-body resistance and aerobic training	Mobility or yoga	Lower-body resistance and aerobic training	Upper-body resistance training with mobility

It's best to avoid physical activities that increase the risk of falling or injury, such as horseback riding or skydiving. Some physical activities are less comfortable and accessible as pregnancy progresses, such as Olympic weightlifting with a barbell, running, or jumping, but this does not necessarily mean those activities are unsafe.

Next, choose which exercises and how many repetitions you want to do. Opt for a repetition range that targets strength endurance, such as 8 to 12 repetitions. Additionally, you can superset strength exercises in a circuit with a stabilization exercise with no rest between exercises. A stabilization exercise can include a single leg or arm exercise or a core-focused exercise. For example, your workout might include 3 rounds of 8 to 12 squats superset with 6 to 10 step-ups per side. This means you would start round 1 with 8 to 12 squats, then perform 6 to 10 step-ups per side, then repeat the circuit with 8 to 12 squats, and so on until all rounds are completed. Squats target lower body strengthening, and pairing them with step-ups emphasizes single-leg stabilization and strength endurance. Finally, you could incorporate a mobility exercise into the circuit, such as a hip or thoracic mobility exercise.

Here is a sample workout using this program design. You'll find other sample workout weeks throughout the book.

SAMPLE PRENATAL WORKOUT

	EXERCISES
Part A	**3 rounds** 10x deadlifts 8x staggered stance Romanian deadlift (RDL) (per side) 5x hip airplanes (per side)
Part B	**3 rounds** 10x bench press 8x diagonal pull-down (per side) 5x thoracic mobility: Cat/cow, side opener, and rotations (per movement)

WORKOUT INTENSITY

There's a misconception that you need to keep your heart rate below a specific target, such as 120 or 140 beats per minute, during pregnancy. But actually, emphasizing your exertion level is more important than your heart rate. Your heart rate can change based on the week of pregnancy, the type of exercise, hydration, age, genetics, and consistency with exercise. Therefore, it doesn't accurately reflect your level of exertion and doesn't serve as a reliable tool to ensure exercise intensity remains "safe." In the first trimester, your heart rate can elevate even with mild exertion, while in the third trimester, your heart rate may sustain a lower rate even with high levels of exertion. It's overall not a reliable measurement.

A more useful way to adjust your workouts is by using the rate of perceived exertion (RPE) scale. RPE is a tool that helps you gauge how hard your exercise feels. Imagine 100 percent as your toughest effort and 0 percent as complete rest. Your RPE can change from day to day because it depends on how you're feeling at that moment. So, don't get caught up in how much weight you're lifting or how fast you're moving. What feels like a 50 percent effort on a Monday might feel like a 70 percent effort on a Thursday. Pay attention to how your body feels on that specific day. This means that you may be lifting lighter weights during pregnancy than you did before or in earlier trimesters. Expect big variations from one day to the next, and be ready to adapt to what your body tells you.

In the first and second trimesters, you can generally exercise at a 70 to 80 percent RPE. As you approach your third trimester, aim for a 50 to 70 percent RPE, as you may find you are generally more fatigued and taxed from pregnancy.

In addition to percentages, you can use an effort level to help you determine what intensity level to seek in your workouts, such as low, moderate, and high. Engaging in exercise across all three effort levels throughout pregnancy is considered safe. The recommended goal is to accumulate 150 minutes of exercise at a moderate intensity per week.

EFFORT FOR PRENATAL WORKOUTS

TRIMESTER	PERCENTAGE FOR WEIGHTS OR EFFORT LEVEL
First	70 to 80 percent RPE*
Second	70 to 80 percent RPE
Third	50 to 70 percent RPE

*RPE = Rate of perceived effort

If you are doing cardio workouts, do the "talk test" to determine which effort level you are exercising. The talk test involves assessing the extent to which you can converse before experiencing breathlessness or requiring a pause in your conversation.

DETERMINING EFFORT LEVEL DURING CARDIO WORKOUTS USING THE TALK TEST

TALK TEST	EFFORT LEVEL
Speak full conversation	Low-intensity level
Speak only a few sentences	Moderate-intensity level
Speak only a few words	High-intensity level

For weightlifting sessions, there are various factors to calibrate your exertion level as either low, moderate, or high intensity. These variables can include adjusting the resistance, repetitions, workout duration, tempo, and rest periods. Increasing and reducing each variable can adjust the overall intensity of the workout, such as increasing weights while decreasing repetitions, or decreasing weights while increasing tempo.

DETERMINING EFFORT LEVEL DURING WEIGHTLIFTING SESSIONS

EFFORT LEVELS	
Too low	Easily completes every repetition, and could do at least 5 to 10 more repetitions before the form is compromised
Moderate	Complete all repetitions with optimal form, but can only do 2 to 3 more repetitions before form becomes compromised
Too high	Either fail the lift or form is compromised during the repetitions

When lifting weights during pregnancy, be sure to maintain near-perfect form for every repetition. Additionally, don't lift weights that are so heavy that you would have to abruptly drop them or sacrifice your form during the set. It's important to maintain optimal form during weightlifting because of the greater joint laxity that comes with pregnancy. This increased joint laxity can make you more vulnerable to injuries if your lifting technique is subpar.

How you approach prenatal workouts is more than selecting a series of pregnancy-safe exercises or omitting "unsafe" exercises. Your prenatal workouts should incorporate elements that support a strong and comfortable pregnancy while preparing you for birth. The next chapters in this section will walk you through these specifics for each trimester.

KEY TAKEAWAYS

The core physical principles of prenatal fitness encompass two fundamental items: alignment and pressure management through breathing strategies. Alignment requires you to be stable in your positions under load, but maintain the ability to change your position in response to movement. By stabilizing the core canister, which comprises the respiratory diaphragm, transverse abdominis, internal oblique muscles, multifidus, and pelvic floor, you establish a solid foundation for movement. This stabilizing framework extends to joint alignment, where stable and rigid joints are contrasted with mobile ones to optimize performance while minimizing the risk of injury.

Recognizing the interplay between intra-abdominal pressure (IAP) and movement demand guides you in adjusting your breathing techniques. The ability to regulate pressure becomes particularly vital during pregnancy, when physical changes may affect your ability to generate high levels of IAP. Adapting your breath-to-movement coordination based on the phases of an exercise—inhaling during lengthening and exhaling during shortening—enhances stability and performance.

FOUR
THE FIRST TRIMESTER

WELCOME TO THE FIRST TRIMESTER! You may have been waiting a few weeks, months, or even years to find yourself in this trimester. So, congratulations! The first trimester can be really exciting at first. You're pregnant! However, this trimester can also be rough, symptoms-wise. Let's delve into how to confidently approach fitness during the first trimester.

Research in the *American Journal of Obstetrics and Gynecology* suggests that moderate-intensity workouts during the first trimester could offer greater advantages compared to waiting until the latter half of your pregnancy. There might be some of us who delay our exercise routines due to concerns about miscarriage. However, it's important to note that this fear is unfounded according to research published in the *British Journal of Sports Medicine* (see chapter 3 for more information). So, don't hesitate to kick-start your exercise routine during the first trimester—it is beneficial for you and your baby (see chapters 1 and 2)!

YOUR PRENATAL WORKOUT ROUTINE

During the first trimester, modifications to movements are primarily driven by early pregnancy symptoms rather than physical limitations. The first trimester is often characterized by a roller coaster of symptoms, from the notorious morning sickness to debilitating fatigue. Navigating these symptoms can be challenging, but they don't necessarily mean the end of your workout routine. Nausea can be managed by opting for smaller, more frequent meals and avoiding exercises that involve lying flat on your back or inverted (upside down). To combat fatigue, prioritize adequate sleep and consider adjusting the intensity and volume of your workouts to suit your energy levels.

If severe nausea makes eating difficult, exercising to burn extra calories is ill-advised and could worsen nausea. Likewise, if fatigue is overwhelming, consider prioritizing more rest during this trimester. You may find that you can't work out during this first trimester, which is okay. In chapter 5, we will discuss how to reintroduce exercise if you need to pause your workouts.

If your pregnancy symptoms are manageable enough to continue working out during this trimester, you may still need to make some modifications to your routine, such as increasing the frequency of rest periods or allowing yourself more time to recover between exercises.

If you are an athlete, you may be used to pushing through discomfort and ignoring signals from your body that suggest you should take it easy or rest. However, pregnancy is not the time to ignore your body's messages and push through discomfort or even pain. On days when fatigue sets in, don't hesitate to decrease the overall volume of your workout. This means reducing the total number of repetitions or sets, allowing your body to conserve energy while staying active.

FIRST-TRIMESTER LIFTING MODIFICATIONS

While the majority of adjustments during the first trimester arise from early pregnancy symptoms, it's possible that as you transition from the end of the first trimester to the start of the second trimester, you may need to modify certain weightlifting routines due to your growing belly. Common modifications include widening the stance for lower body movements to make more space for your belly. This is particularly relevant when hip flexion becomes uncomfortable due to the belly pressing against the thigh. For movements like the deadlift, opt for a wider or sumo stance.

Another modification aimed at creating room for your developing baby involves elevating the bar to reduce the range of motion at the bottom part of the exercise, thereby decreasing hip flexion. For instance, in exercises like the deadlift or hip thrust, raising the bar using boxes or bumper plates can limit the extent to which the bar needs to be lowered. This adjustment can allow you to sustain a traditional deadlift stance and, in the case of the hip thrust, facilitate more comfortable positioning beneath the bar. This modification minimizes the pressure of the bar between the abdomen and thighs at the point of maximum hip flexion during the hip thrust.

COMMON FIRST-TRIMESTER LIFTING MODIFICATIONS

MOVEMENT	MODIFICATIONS
Deadlift	Elevated deadlift with conventional stance Wider or sumo stance
Hip thrust	Elevated hip thrust
Pull-ups	Banded pull-ups Lat pull-down
Bench press	Feet elevated on bench Inclined (nausea or heartburn)

As you near the end of the first trimester, you might also observe abdominal coning during core-focused exercises, including pull-ups, or movements involving abdominal flexion, such as sit-ups. (Abdominal coning is when the center of the abdomen pushes out further than the rest of the abdominal wall.) You can modify pull-ups by using resistance bands to decrease overall exertion or transition to lat pull-downs with either bands or a cable machine. If coning arises with abdominal flexion, prioritize exercises that involve anti-rotation or rotational movements, as discussed in depth on page 60 of this chapter.

SAMPLE FIRST-TRIMESTER WORKOUT

In the following sample first-trimester workout, all exercises maintain an upright position, with rest periods between sets. This workout has been condensed to two rounds and has reduced repetitions for each exercise. This is just an example of how you could modify your first-trimester workouts.

COMMON FIRST-TRIMESTER CONCERNS

For many of my prenatal clients, the common first-trimester concerns revolve around symptoms affecting their workout routine and which exercises are "safe" for pregnancy. Because of the overwhelmingly negative beliefs about prenatal exercise, you may feel that you have this very long list of "unsafe" exercises to avoid, but not a very robust list of exercises that are safe and beneficial for you. In this

SAMPLE FIRST TRIMESTER WORKOUT

	LOWER BODY WORKOUT	UPPER BODY WORKOUT
WARM-UP	Seated breathing drill 90/90 side opener	Standing back expansion Forward lat release
WORKOUT	**A: 2 to 3 rounds** 10x elevated deadlift 8x single-leg deadlift with banded row 5x hip airplanes **B: 2 to 3 rounds** 10x elevated hip thrust 8x standing fire hydrants 20 seconds Copenhagen plank **C: 2 rounds** 10x crossover step-up 30x lateral band walk	**A: 2 to 3 rounds** 10x bench press (incline or feet elevated) 8x diagonal pull-down 10x one-sided carry standing marches (per side) **B: 2 to 3 rounds** 10x banded pull-ups or pull-downs 8x overhead tricep extensions 10x banded pull-aparts **C: 2 to 3 rounds** 5x standing keg lift 10x snow angels Seated thoracic mobility

section, I will discuss how you can manage common first-trimester symptoms that may make working out difficult, and how to approach core training in pregnancy, which is commonly believed to be "unsafe."

FIRST-TRIMESTER SYMPTOMS: NAUSEA AND FATIGUE

The most common symptoms in the first trimester are nausea, which may or may not include vomiting, and extreme fatigue. The combination of these symptoms may make it challenging to continue a substantial workout routine in the first trimester. If you do find that exercising makes your symptoms worse, it is okay—you can resume workouts in the second trimester when you feel better. In my own pregnancies, my workout routine drastically decreased in frequency due to nausea and fatigue. It can be ideal to honor that you need more rest in these early weeks. Remember, you are doing a lot in these beginning weeks of pregnancy—you are growing a whole human being, which is incredible, so it is okay to rest if you need to.

If you do find that you can continue to work out, go for it! You may find that maintaining a more upright position helps to relieve nausea, and incorporating longer rest periods between exercises helps to manage your fatigue levels. Additionally, you can decrease the overall length of your workout to accommodate your energy levels, which may be lower in the first trimester.

CORE TRAINING

There's a pervasive myth that all core exercises should be avoided during pregnancy because they could damage your core and make abdominal separation, or *diastasis recti abdominis* (DRA), worse (see page 61 for more on abdominal separation). Let's debunk this right now. A strong core that can both contract and lengthen is necessary during pregnancy to accommodate changes in your musculoskeletal system and to support your baby's position in preparation for birth. You can continue to do core exercises in the first trimester and throughout your entire pregnancy. However, not every core exercise is appropriate for pregnancy. In this section, I will break down how you can tell whether an exercise is appropriate for you and when you should modify or omit specific core exercises.

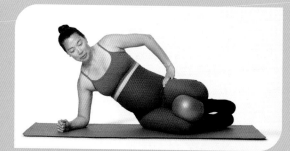
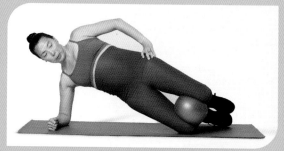

SIDE-LYING HIP ABDUCTION WITH BALL SQUEEZE

The side-lying hip abduction is a core stabilization exercise that strengthens the obliques and glutes. Think of this movement as doing a sideways glute bridge—the hips will move forward to extend, not lift directly upward to the ceiling.

1 Start in a side-lying position, with your elbow, hip, and ankle in a straight line, with your knees bent in front of you.

2 Place a soft object, like an exercise ball, between your knees.

3 Exhale to push the hips forward, simultaneously squeezing the ball between your knees.

4 Inhale to sit the hips back into the starting position.

5 Repeat 5 to 10 times per side.

You can make this movement more challenging by omitting the ball between the knees, adding a ball balance, or adding in a chest press (see variations). Be sure to maintain the same movement pattern in the advanced exercises.

First, let's define what a core exercise is, because core exercises are more than just sit-ups and crunches. Core exercises target the muscles of the torso to either resist movement, support the spine's movement, or move the spine itself. Let's look at each in turn.

Core Exercises That Resist Motion

When your core is resisting motion, you are maintaining your torso's position as your arms and legs move. This allows your extremities to anchor off your core to complete functional movement, such as squats, where you are limiting how much your torso moves as you bend and extend your legs. Side-lying hip abduction and bird dog are other examples.

Variation 1: Side-Lying Hip Abduction with Ball Balance
In this exercise, a Pilates ball is placed under the bottom knee to decrease the stability and increase the activation of the core.

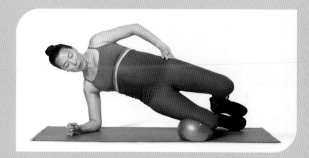

Variation 2: Side-Lying Hip Abduction with Banded Chest Press
In this exercise, the top arm is pressing a band forward as the hip simultaneously extends.

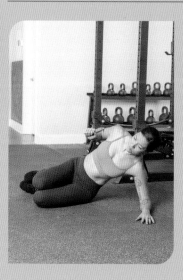

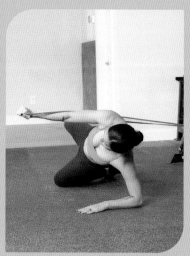

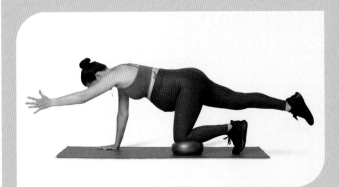

BIRD DOG BALANCE

The bird dog is another core stabilization exercise that strengthens the abdominal muscles and glutes. Similar to the side-lying hip abduction, you can make this exercise more challenging by placing a ball under the support knee. This increases the instability of the exercise to further strengthen the core and hip muscles.

1 Start in a tabletop position.

2 Exhale to reach one arm forward as you extend the opposite leg backward.

3 As you extend the arm and leg, maintain your torso position and avoid arching in the back.

4 Inhale to return to the starting position.

Two cues may be helpful:

- **Imagine you are trying to stand** on the wall behind you, not lifting your foot toward the ceiling. Lifting the foot toward the ceiling will cause you to arch in your back, which would remove the core stabilization aspect of this exercise.
- **As you extend, focus on** maintaining the same distance between the rib cage and pelvis on the front side of the body throughout the entire movement.

    You can make the bird dog more challenging by incorporating a weight or resistance band, such as with a banded pull-down or weighted row.

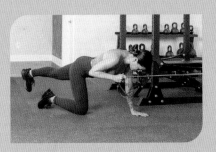

Variation 1: Bird Dog with Banded Pull-Down
In this core exercise, you will straighten one leg to activate the glute as you pull down a band with the opposite arm to activate the lat muscle. In addition to being a prenatal-safe core exercise, this exercise targets the posterior oblique sling that stabilizes the lower back and back pelvic joints.

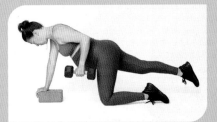

Variation 2: Bird Dog with Weighted Row
In this tabletop core exercise, as you extend one leg backward to activate the glute, you will row a weight with the opposite arm. Placing the support hand on a yoga block or holding another dumbbell increases the range of motion of the moving arm.

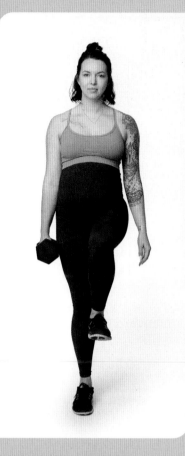

BRIDGE MARCHES WITH OVERHEAD RESISTANCE

This exercise is another anti-extension movement that can be a modification from the sit-up or other abdominal flexion core exercises. In this movement, you resist arching your back in the bridge position while maintaining a pull-down as your legs move.

1 Start in a supine position with a band attached overhead.

2 Pull the band so your hands are over your shoulders, ensuring there is still tension in the band. You should feel like you are resisting a pull toward the point of attachment.

3 Elevate the hips into a bridge position.

4 Maintain your hip and torso position as you lift one foot off the ground.

5 Switch legs.

6 Repeat for 5 to 10 repetitions per side.

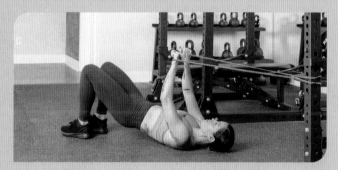

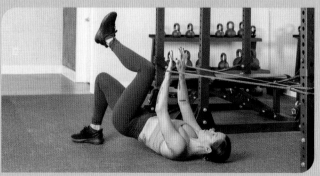

FARMER CARRY

In the farmer carry, you are resisting lateral flexion, or bending, in the side of your body. In this move-ment, you can hold weights in both hands, different weights in each hand, or different positions such as suitcase and front rack, or only one weight. These carrying variations can challenge the core in different ways. In the farmer carry, you will maintain your torso position as you walk or march in place.

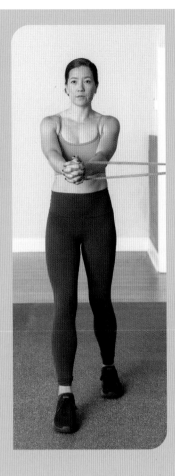
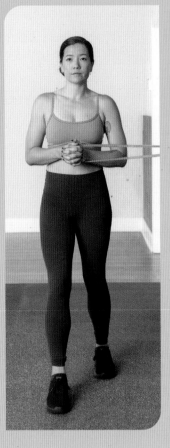

PALLOF PRESS

This is an anti-rotation exercise, where you are resisting a pull laterally. You have the option to keep your feet parallel, stagger the stance, or find a more supportive position, such as seated, kneeling, or supine.

1 Stand perpendicular to the point of attachment and bring the band into the center of your chest. You should feel a pull toward the point of attachment.

2 Exhale to press the band outward, as you keep it aligned to the center of your chest. The pull should increase as your hands move away from your body.

3 Inhale to bring the band back in.

4 Repeat 5 to 10 times and switch sides.

Core Exercises That Move the Spine

Core exercises that focus on changing the spine's position can include movements that cause the spine to:

- Curl or round and extend, such as crunches or sit-ups
- Laterally bend and extend, such as side crunches
- Rotate or twist, such as Russian twists

However, traditional core exercises, like crunches, side crunches, or Russian twists, may not be appropriate for pregnancy. These exercises tend to isolate the abdominal muscles, which is not usually helpful for pregnancy when you want your core to work in unison with the upper and lower body. When your core works in synchronization with the rest of your body, it can improve stability and decrease common aches and pains associated with pregnancy. Additionally, these exercises tend to cause abdominal coning, which is a symptom showing that the core exercise is no longer beneficial and could be damaging to the abdominal wall (see below).

ABDOMINAL SEPARATION (DIASTASIS)

Abdominal separation, or DRA, is a normal and necessary feature of pregnancy. Abdominal separation is when the connective tissue down the center of the belly stretches and thins to accommodate your baby's growth. You cannot prevent diastasis, but you can minimize the severity by being aware of how you are moving your body and what type of core exercises you are incorporating into your prenatal workout routine.

One major symptom to be aware of during your workouts, especially core-focused exercises, is abdominal coning. Abdominal coning is when the center of the abdomen pushes out further than the rest of the abdominal wall. This occurs due to the connective tissue being thinner than the surrounding muscles and more easily manipulated by changes in pressure. When there is too much intra-abdominal pressure (IAP), and the abdominal wall cannot counter the increased pressure, this center connective tissue pushes out further, causing abdominal coning. Coning may look like a tent or linear bump down the center of the abdomen.

However, not all abdominal coning is something to panic about—if you are just relaxing and your abdomen forms a cone, it is generally not an issue. This is known as a *soft cone*, where there is no internal pressure pushing against the connective tissue, but rather just how your abs are relaxing. Abdominal coning is an issue if the coning occurs under exertion, such as when exercising, and is a "hard cone," firm to touch. This type of coning is caused by an increase in IAP pushing out against this connective tissue. If the connective tissue is repeatedly being stretched and manipulated by changes in pressure, it could damage the tissue more than normal. This increased damage can worsen abdominal separation and make it harder to heal after birth.

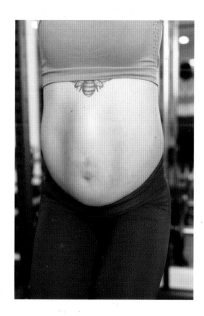

How can you minimize or alleviate abdominal coning? First, you can focus on maintaining a neutral spine position, rather than arching in the back during movement. In an arched position, the connective tissue of the abdominal wall is stretched and thinned more than usual, and it is more easily manipulated by pressure changes.

Second, you can adjust the equipment, adjust your setup from standing to seated or half kneeling, or adjust the angle of a movement.

Common exercises that cause coning are:

- Overhead press (as shown)
- Vertical pulling exercises: Pull-ups
- Core intensive exercises: Planks
- Abdominal flexion exercises: Sit-ups, crunches, V-ups

If you are experiencing abdominal coning, choose one of the modifications for each exercise group detailed below that allows you to continue to accomplish that movement pattern without coning. The modification variation you need will likely continue to change throughout your pregnancy. Let's look at modifications for each of these exercises.

Modifications for Overhead Press

The overhead press is one of the most common exercises that can cause abdominal coning. As you press weight overhead, there may be a tendency to arch your back to shift the effort from the shoulders to the chest. This compensation pattern can occur due to poor positioning at the start of the exercise, the weight being too heavy, or restriction in shoulder mobility. Let's look at some ways to modify if you notice coning in the overhead press.

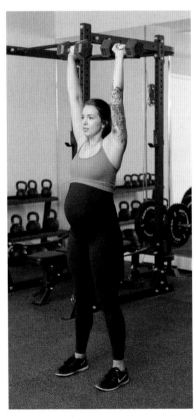

BARBELL TO DUMBBELL MODIFICATION: For the overhead press, the first modification is to change from using a barbell to dumbbells. When you use a barbell to press overhead, you must clear the bar path by either shifting the bar forward or your body backward. Eventually, to accomplish this shift, you will need to arch the spine, which can cause abdominal coning. Transitioning to dumbbells alleviates the need to shift your position to clear the bar path, which can resolve coning.

STANDING TO SEATED MODIFICATION: The next modification is to adjust your setup from a standing position, which requires more stabilization, to a seated position, which is more supportive. In a seated position, add a wedge or support under the back half of your hips to help maintain a neutral position. Then, you can add a Pilates ball or soft object between your knees to activate your inner thighs, which can increase the activation of your pelvic floor and core musculature. Increased

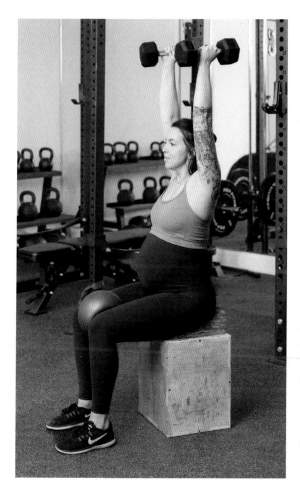
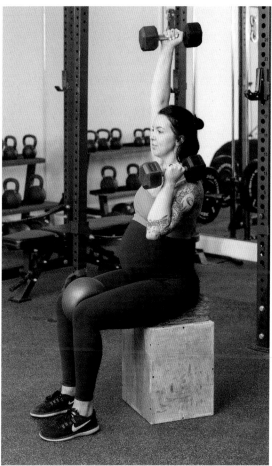

activation of the deep core increases the thickness of the abdominal wall, which can prevent coning.

In this supported position, the most difficult variation is pressing two weights overhead at the same time, followed by alternating the weights overhead. The easiest is a single-arm overhead press, which allows you to use your free hand to provide external feedback and monitor your rib positioning. Choose a variation that allows you to monitor your form and minimize abdominal coning.

If you are still having trouble with coning during the overhead press even with the previous modifications, you can continue to modify by adding external feedback in the opposite direction or adjusting the angle of the press from overhead to about a 45-degree angle. Both of these modifications can help you maintain a more neutral spine position to prevent coning.

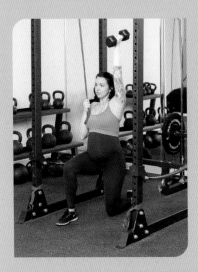

HALF-KNEELING PULL-DOWN WITH OVERHEAD PRESS

This exercise modification includes using external feedback in the opposite direction to help you maintain your neutral rib position. In the half-kneeling position, grab a band overhead with the hand of the forward leg and pull it down toward your torso. This will engage your core to keep the rib cage down to alleviate coning. Maintain the downward pull on the band as you press and lower the weight.

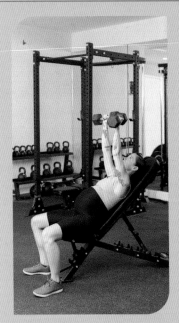

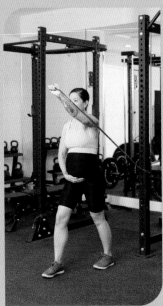

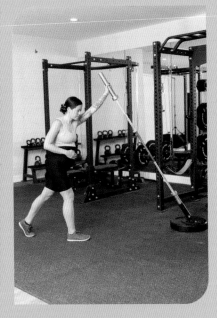

INCLINE PRESS: DUMBBELLS AND BANDED AND LANDMINE PRESS

This exercise modification strategy involves adjusting the press angle from directly overhead to about a 45-degree angle. Sometimes you can't press weight directly overhead without arching due to shoulder or upper back (thoracic) mobility limitations. Instead, you can decrease the pressing angle to a point that is accessible to alleviate the tendency to arch as you press overhead and minimize abdominal coning. You can accomplish this by using an incline dumbbell bench press, an incline banded press, or a landmine press.

Modifications for Vertical Pull

Similar to overhead pressing exercises, vertical pulling exercises can be a common reason for abdominal coning due to the tendency to arch the back during the exercise. If you are experiencing coning with exercises where you are pulling a weight from overhead to your body, such as pull-ups or lat pull-downs, there are a number of modifications you can try to improve your positioning and prevent coning.

BANDED PULL-UPS: VERTICAL AND HORIZONTAL SETUPS

The first modification strategy for vertically pulling movements, such as the pull-up, includes utilizing more bands to make the movement more accessible. You may experience coning with pull-ups if the movement is too challenging, so incorporating the bands can decrease your effort while allowing you to maintain the overall movement pattern. There are two options to set up the bands for the banded pull-ups.

In one variation, the band is attached vertically to the pull-up bar. This is the most common setup, but could result in a lot of swinging that may alter your position, causing abdominal coning.

The second variation is a horizontal band setup. This requires a power rack with j-hooks to attach the band horizontally, so there may be equipment limitations. You will stand on the band to do your banded pull-ups, which results in significantly less swinging and can improve your overall positioning to prevent coning.

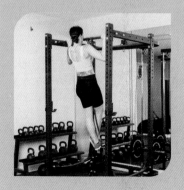
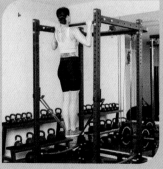

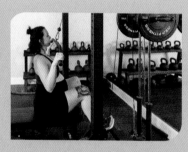

LAT PULL-DOWN

If the banded variation is not accessible for you, either due to equipment or if you are still experiencing coning even with banded support, a lat pull-down with a cable machine or band can be a great alternative. When doing a lat pull-down, avoid arching your back as you pull the bar toward your chest. Additionally, you can bend more at your hips by placing your feet on an elevated surface in front of you, which can decrease the effort in your core. You can also squeeze a ball between your thighs to increase activation of your pelvic floor and abdominal wall to increase the thickness of the muscles to prevent coning.

If all vertical pulling exercises and their modifications are still causing abdominal coning, modifying to a horizontal pulling exercise, such as bent-over rows (page 126) or single-arm dumbbell rows (page 101) can be a great option. These exercises are still similarly strengthening the back musculature and are a valuable alternative during pregnancy.

Modifications for Core Intensive Exercises: Planks

Core intensive exercises, particularly ones that emphasize isometric holds like the plank, can cause abdominal coning due to being simply too challenging during pregnancy. You could continue to plank for several months into your pregnancy, but eventually, you may notice that your core begins to cone. If you begin to experience coning, you can increase the elevation of the plank by placing your hands on a bench or chair, which can decrease the intensity of the exercise. You can also modify from a plank to a bear position to decrease the intensity of the exercise.

PALLOF PRESS WITH ROTATIONS

The Pallof press with rotation incorporates the anti-rotation from the previous section and then adds on the rotational element to strengthen the obliques.

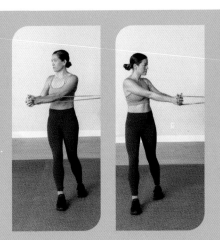

1 Repeat steps 1 to 2 of the Pallof press (page 60).

2 Continue to exhale as you rotate away from the point of attachment.

3 Inhale to return to the starting position.

4 Repeat 5 to 10 times and switch sides.

Modifications for Abdominal Flexion: Sit-Ups and Crunches

Core exercises that emphasize abdominal flexion, crunching, and curling up in the abs can cause abdominal coning. Abdominal flexion exercises tend to target the six-pack abs. During pregnancy, crunchlike exercises can overactivate the six-pack abs and deactivate the deep core muscles, which causes abdominal coning.

In lieu of abdominal flexion exercises, you can incorporate core exercises that focus on a different direction of movement, such as rotational core exercises.

BEAR POSITION PLANK

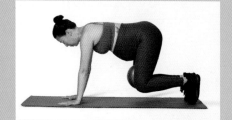

If the banded variation is not accessible for you, either due to equipment or if you are still experiencing coning even with banded support, a lat pull-down with a cable machine or band can be a great alternative. When doing a lat pull-down, avoid arching your back as you pull the bar toward your chest. Additionally, you can bend more at your hips by placing your feet on an elevated surface in front of you, which can decrease the effort in your core. You can also squeeze a ball between your thighs to increase activation of your pelvic floor and abdominal wall to increase the thickness of the muscles to prevent coning.

Rotational core exercises strengthen the oblique muscles and can have a positive effect on managing abdominal separation during pregnancy and healing it after birth. Movements that involve rotation include Pallof rotations, described above. There are more rotational core exercises in chapter 5 on page 79.

Diastasis is a normal part of pregnancy—there is nothing you can do to prevent abdominal separation, as it needs to happen to accommodate your baby's growth. But you can decrease the severity of diastasis by being aware of any abdominal coning with exertion. If you are exercising, particularly with vertical pressing or pulling movements, and you experience abdominal coning, find a modification that allows you to still accomplish the intent of the exercise in a way that accommodates your current core capabilities.

KEY TAKEAWAYS

During the first trimester, there are usually not a lot of physical modifications in your exercises. Most exercises will closely resemble your prepregnancy routine, but you may need to make adjustments because of energy levels or nausea. There may be some modifications required toward the end of the first trimester as your belly grows and certain lifts become uncomfortable. Now, let's transition to discussing the second trimester!

FIVE
THE SECOND TRIMESTER

AS YOU TRANSITION INTO THE SECOND TRIMESTER, you may notice an uptick in energy levels, and your physical appearance might start to reflect your pregnancy. However, it's important to recognize that the visible signs of pregnancy may not become fully apparent until the third trimester for some individuals, and that's perfectly normal. The size of your belly can be influenced by numerous factors unrelated to your overall health or the well-being of your baby.

Be aware that regardless of the reasons, you're likely to receive an increase in comments about your size during this period. These comments could range from concerns about being too large to comments about your belly being too small. It's a common phenomenon during pregnancy that people tend to offer unsolicited advice, which can be unwelcome and intrusive.

In the second trimester, you'll probably need to start modifying your exercises to accommodate your growing belly. You may also begin to suffer from common prenatal discomforts, such as lower back or pelvic girdle pain. There is a common belief that pelvic girdle pain and other ailments are normal and acceptable parts of pregnancy, and that there is nothing you can do to overcome these discomforts. This is completely untrue! In this chapter, we will thoroughly debunk this idea and discuss specific strategies to overcome pelvic girdle pain.

SECOND-TRIMESTER LIFTING MODIFICATIONS

The main modifications in this trimester focus on making space for your belly by widening your stance and decreasing hip flexion at the bottom of lower body exercises, similar to the end of the first trimester. For example, changing from a conventional deadlift to a sumo deadlift.

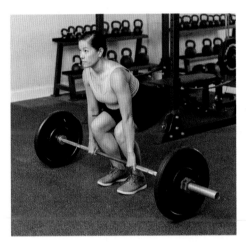
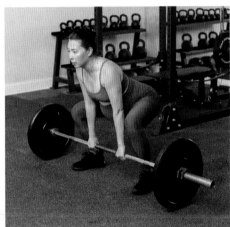

Another common modification toward the end of the first trimester into the early second trimester is to elevate your feet to the same level as your body while doing supine exercises, such as the bench press. The reason for this modification is that as pregnancy advances, the increased curvature of the lower back can be uncomfortable to maintain if your feet are on the floor during a bench press.

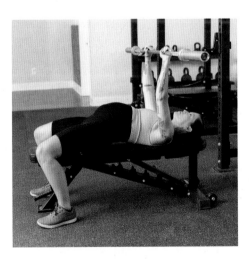
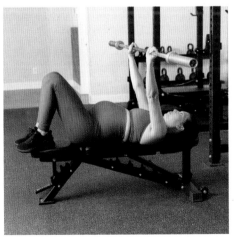

COMMON SECOND TRIMESTER MODIFICATIONS

MOVEMENT	MODIFICATIONS
Squat	Wider stances Back squats Box squats
Deadlift	Wider or sumo stance Elevated barbell with conventional lift Elevated barbell with sumo stance
Hip thrust	Elevated hip thrust Elevated hip thrust with Fat Gripz Dumbbell hip thrust Banded hip thrust (horizontal setup)
Bench press (horizontal push)	Feet elevated bench press
Pull-up (vertical pull)	Banded pull-ups (vertical or horizontal band) Cable pull-down Straight-arm pull-down
Rows (horizontal pull)	Bent-over row Single-arm row with support
Overhead press (vertical push)	Barbell overhead press Dumbbell overhead press Seated overhead press Half kneeling press with banded pull-down

Additionally, you may begin to include more support in your lifts, such as box squats or seated variations of upper body exercises. If you have pelvic girdle pain or pain with single leg movements, find a modification that does not cause pain (descriptions of these modifications follow). During this trimester, you may also find that higher-impact activities like running or jumping are no longer comfortable, so you may opt to transition to stationary cardio machines, such as a stationary bike or rower, or low-impact aerobic activity like swimming.

SAMPLE SECOND-TRIMESTER WORKOUT

Use the following workout template as a guide for your second-trimester workouts or develop your own using the exercises listed throughout this chapter. If you took your first trimester off due to nausea and fatigue (the first trimester is just rough sometimes), you may need to ease back into workouts. I do not recommend rushing back to a prepregnancy level of intensity once you feel energized again; rather, start with a workout that lasts 15 to 20 minutes, and gradually add on time until you reach your desired training duration. You'll find that you can usually resume your desired workout volume and intensity levels within 2 weeks.

With this sample workout, if you are resuming workouts in the second trimester, you may opt for two rounds instead of three to decrease the workout volume. Additionally, you should resume workouts at 50- to 70-percent intensity levels and gradually return to 70- to 90-percent intensity over the 2- to 3-week period.

SAMPLE SECOND-TRIMESTER WORKOUT

	LOWER BODY WORKOUT	UPPER BODY WORKOUT
WARM-UP	Sacroiliac joint dysfunction (SJD) reset exercise Seated side opener	Pubic symphysis dysfunction (SPD) reset exercise Adductor rock back (right side)
WORKOUT	**A: 3 rounds** 10x elevated hip thrust 8x lateral step-up with banded row 5x hip airplanes **B: 2 to 3 rounds** 10x elevated Romanian deadlift (RDL) 20x lateral band walk (or modification) **C: 3 rounds** 10x Bulgarian split squat 30 second Copenhagen plank 5x hip airplane 20- to 30-minute walk	**A: 3 rounds** 10x seated dumbbell strict press 10x side-lying hip abduction 5x thoracic mobility **B: 3 rounds** 10x bent-over row 8x diagonal banded pull-down 10x pull apart **C: 3 rounds** 10x single-arm dumbbell row 6x bear position pass throughs 20- to 30-minute walk

COMMON SECOND-TRIMESTER CONCERNS: PELVIC GIRDLE PAIN

As you navigate the second trimester, in addition to resuming exercise if you paused workouts in your first trimester due to nausea and fatigue, you may begin to experience some sort of pelvic girdle pain. This could be due to lots of physical changes happening in this trimester as your belly grows and your center of gravity shifts. Additionally, a lack of exercise contributed to a period of deconditioning that has made it harder for you to stabilize your pelvic joints. This pelvic pain can range from mild to debilitating, making even walking incredibly painful. In this section, I will define pelvic girdle pain, explain what causes it, and present several solutions for a pain-free pregnancy. Remember, pain is not a requirement of pregnancy.

One of the more prevalent second (and third) trimester complaints is pelvic girdle pain. Pelvic girdle pain can be characterized by sharp, sudden pain in the front of the pelvis, groin, and upper inner thigh, known as *pubic symphysis dysfunction,* or SPD. Pelvic girdle pain can also present as deep pain within the gluteal area at the back of the pelvis or lower back, known as *sacroiliac joint dysfunction,* or SJD. You may not initially recognize this as pelvic girdle pain. Some might refer to it as sciatic pain, especially if it's felt more in the back or deep within the gluteal region. Others might associate it with lower back pain, while some could simply be unsure about its nature. It's pelvic girdle pain if the pain worsens when doing single-leg exercises or making pivoting movements, such as walking, changing direction, exiting a vehicle, or shifting position in bed.

If you're experiencing pelvic girdle pain, you may have been told that the only way to find relief is to give birth. This was the only solution presented to me when I discussed my pelvic girdle pain with my provider during my first pregnancy. Or you may believe pelvic pain is a normal and unpreventable part of pregnancy and not seek additional care. This is far from true! To begin with, pelvic girdle pain doesn't necessarily vanish immediately after birth and in fact can continue for several months after giving birth.

Pelvic girdle pain is typically caused by one or a combination of two primary factors: pelvic asymmetry and biomechanical patterns. While some might assume that the hormone relaxin contributes to pelvic pain due to heightened joint flexibility, research published in the *European Spine Journal* has discredited this notion: Elevated relaxin levels do not align with an increased occurrence of pelvic girdle pain.

Note that neither reason is pregnancy—pregnancy does not cause pelvic girdle pain; however, pregnancy may exaggerate preexisting movement patterns and asymmetry that could contribute to pelvic pain. Without addressing and rectifying the positioning of the pelvis and underlying biomechanical issues, pelvic girdle pain may persist for several months postpartum.

PELVIC ASYMMETRY

Pelvic asymmetry refers to the positioning of the two halves of the pelvic girdle, which are connected by pelvic joints. The front of the pelvic girdle is linked by the pubic symphysis joint, while the back connects to the sacrum—the triangular bone located at the rear of the pelvis—through the sacroiliac joints. Pelvic asymmetry is when these two pelvic halves are not well aligned, typically resulting in the left half rotating forward and the right half rotating backward.

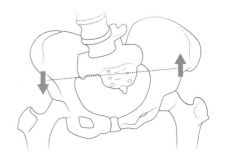

The pelvic girdle is designed to allow slight movement during physical activity. As you walk and maneuver your body, one half of the pelvic girdle rotates forward while the other moves backward. During this motion, the pelvic joints should come together closely to provide stabilization, known as *form closure,* where the joints fit snugly together to create stability. If a joint lacks proper alignment, achieving form closure can become challenging, potentially leading to heightened movement or even a shearing motion within the joint, resulting in discomfort.

The pelvis is connected to various muscles that influence its position. If certain muscles are significantly more active than their opposing counterparts, it can cause an imbalanced torque or pull on the pelvis. A common scenario involves the shortening of the left hip flexor and quadriceps muscles and the right hamstring and adductor muscles. This uneven pull leads to the left half of the pelvis tilting forward and the right half tilting backward, creating an asymmetrical pelvic position. However, it's important to note that the pelvis is naturally designed for movement. The issue arises when the muscular equilibrium required to pull the pelvis into the counterbalancing position—with the right hip forward and the left hip backward—is absent.

If your pain is arising from pelvic asymmetry, there are several strategies to improve the pelvic position, including physical resetting of the pelvic position with exercises or chiropractic adjustments, mobility exercises to release the uneven pull on the pelvis, and strengthening exercises to counteract the imbalanced muscular pull on the pelvis. I cover each below.

Pelvic Resetting Exercises

Pelvic resetting exercises focus on two specific joints: the pubic symphysis joint, which is situated at the front of the pelvis, and the sacroiliac joints, which are located at the back of the pelvis.

FRONT OF PELVIS RESET EXERCISE

The initial reset exercise focuses on the front pelvic joint. To perform this exercise, you'll need to be in a seated position and have a ball or soft object to hold between your knees. This exercise offers four distinct variations. In the first variation, align your feet parallel to each other with your toes facing forward. In the second variation, angle your feet outward at approximately 45 degrees. For the third variation, angle your feet inward at roughly 45 degrees.

In the fourth variation, the left hip shifts backward as the right hip shifts forward because the common positioning of the pelvis is the opposite, with the left hip forward and the right hip backward. If the pelvic pain is due to pelvic positioning, the hip shift in this direction can release tension that can make it easier to change the position of your pelvis to support stabilization as you walk and move.

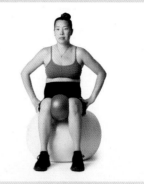

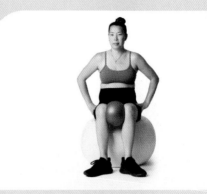

1 Begin in a seated position; place a ball or soft object between your knees.

2 Start with the setup for variation 1, with your feet parallel, and then proceed to variation 2, with your toes pointed outward; 3, with your toes pointed inward; and 4, hip shift with the left hip shifted backward and right hip shifting forward, using the following guidelines for each variation.

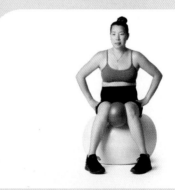

3 Inhale deeply, expanding your rib cage and back. You'll notice an increased pressure in the pelvic floor during inhalation.

4 Exhale as you squeeze the ball between your knees gently, simultaneously lifting the pelvic floor.

5 Inhale to release tension on the ball.

6 Repeat this sequence a total of 10 times.

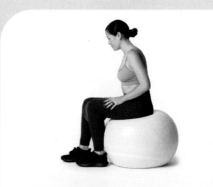

BACK OF PELVIS RESET EXERCISE

The next reset exercise targets the joints at the back of the pelvis. Choose a progression of this movement that feels comfortable for you. To perform this exercise, you'll need a yoga block or a raised surface 2 to 3 inches (5–8 cm) in height.

1 Begin in a tabletop position, with the left knee elevated on a yoga block.

2 Shift your weight toward the left knee, which should result in a more noticeable stretch in the left glute. If you find it challenging to shift your weight toward the left knee, press the right knee against a wall to help move your weight over the left knee. Make sure the right knee remains lower than the height of the block.

3 Push the belly away from the floor to find a rounding in the back.

4 Hold this position and take 10 full breaths.

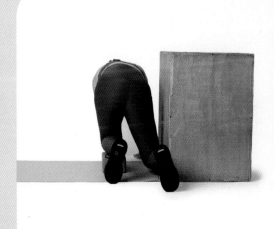

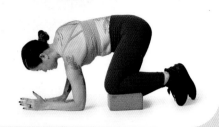

Continuing: Variation 1

1 While maintaining the hip-shifted table-top position, lower your left forearm to the floor.

2 You should feel a compression on the left side of the body.

3 Keep pushing your belly away from the floor to sustain the rounded back posture.

4 Hold this position and take 10 full breaths.

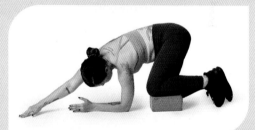

Continuing: Variation 2

1 Keeping your left forearm on the floor, extend your right arm forward and place it in front of your left hand.

2 You should feel a stretch on the right side of the body.

3 Keep pushing your belly away from the floor to sustain the rounded back posture.

4 Hold this position and take 10 full breaths.

Mobility Exercises

Another strategy to reset the pelvic position includes releasing the muscles responsible for pulling the pelvis into this rotated position. In many cases, the left hip flexors and quadriceps and the right adductors (inner thigh muscles) need to be released.

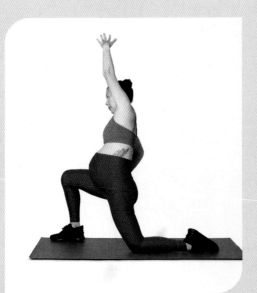

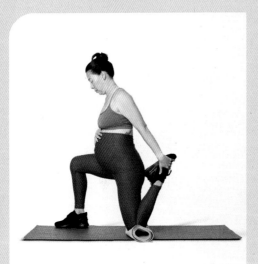

HIP AND QUAD RELEASE

The muscles that pull the pelvis forward are the hip flexors and quadricep muscles. Often, these muscles are shortened on the left side compared to the right. Releasing tension in the left hip flexor and quadriceps can assist in rotating the left half of the pelvis backward, supporting a more symmetrical pelvic position.

1 Begin in a half kneeling position, with the left knee down and right left forward.

2 Tuck the butt underneath. You should feel more of a stretch in the front side of the left hip.

3 Push the hips forward while maintaining this tucked hip position. This should intensify the stretch in the front side of the hip.

4 Extend the left arm up toward the ceiling and then reach toward the right side. You should feel a stretch through the left side of the body.

5 Maintain this position for 10 breaths.

6 Reach behind you to grasp the left foot with one or both hands.

7 Pull the foot toward your glutes to feel a stretch in the front side of the left thigh.

8 Maintain this position for 10 breaths.

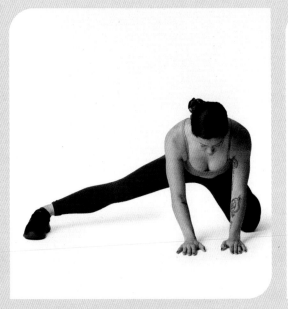

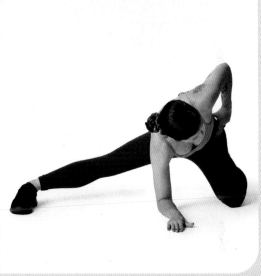

ADDUCTOR ROCK BACK

The muscles that pull the pelvis backward with internal rotation are the adductors (inner thigh muscles) and hamstrings. Often, these muscles are shortened on the right side compared to the left. Releasing tension in the right adductor can allow the right half of the pelvis to rotate forward with external rotation.

1 Begin with your left knee on the ground and your left ankle behind you in a half kneeling position.

2 Extend the right leg straight out to the side. You should feel more of a stretch in the inner right thigh and groin area.

3 Shift your weight back toward the left heel. This will increase the stretch in your right inner thigh.

4 Increase the stretch of this posture by dropping the right elbow to the floor, which will facilitate the rotation of your upper body.

5 Hold this position for 10 breaths or perform a rocking motion back and forth for 10 repetitions.

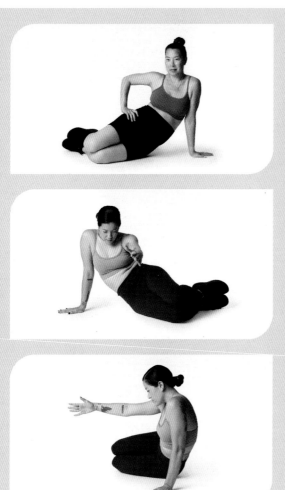

SIDE OPENER

Limitations in rib cage mobility affect pelvic mobility. When dealing with asymmetry, it's crucial to look beyond the immediate pain area. Often, there's increased compression on the right side of the rib cage. To encourage a more balanced pelvic position, you'll focus on expanding the side of the body.

1 In a side seated position, let the ribs and side of your body fall toward the floor. You should feel a stretching sensation in the side of your body toward the floor.

2 Then reach forward with the top arm as you push the chest away from the hand to round in the back.

3 Hold the position for 5 to 10 breaths, then switch sides.

Strengthening Exercises

The final approach to addressing pelvic asymmetry incorporates strengthening exercises. Muscles can only pull, not push, so if you are trying to correct the pelvic position, you need to also focus on strengthening the muscles that are over-lengthened in addition to stretching. If you favor a right stance, focus on strengthening the right glute and quad and the left adductor and hamstring. If you favor a bilateral stance, focus on strengthening the adductor and hamstring on both sides.

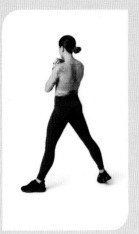
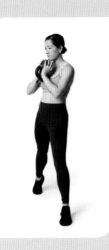

SPLIT SQUAT WITH INTERNAL AND EXTERNAL ROTATION

Pelvic girdle pain can be due to limited hip mobility. In single-leg exercises, such as the split squat or lunge, you can increase rotation at the hip to strengthen the glute, enhance hip mobility, and improve pelvic positioning.

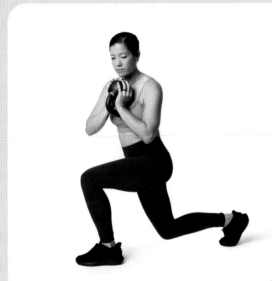

1 Start in the split squat stance with one leg forward and the other leg behind you.

2 Inhale to lower to the bottom of your split squat, while rotating your belly toward your thigh to find internal rotation. If you are having trouble finding internal rotation at the bottom, you can bring the back knee behind your front leg to emphasize this rotation.

3 Maintain the alignment of your front knee over the ankle throughout the entire movement. Keeping weight in the big toe of the forward leg can help maintain this alignment and could increase the activation of the glute.

4 At the bottom of this movement, you will feel more of a stretching sensation in the glute and hamstring of the forward leg.

5 Exhale to extend in the legs, while rotating your belly outward to find external rotation.

6 At the top of this movement, you should feel more of a contraction in the glute and stretching sensation in the forward leg groin.

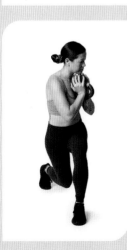
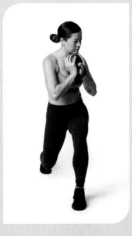

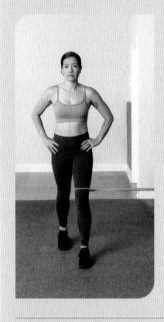

BANDED LATERAL RESISTANCE

Sometimes pelvic pain is due to decreased activation of the supporting muscles, such as when the right glute or left adductor just don't fire enough to help with stability. You can incorporate a resistance band to provide some external feedback to help these muscles turn on a bit more, a strategy that you might find helps relieve pelvic pain almost instantly!

The following exercises use resistance bands to modify the direction of pull, focusing on either adduction—bringing the legs closer together—to primarily strengthen the adductors, or abduction—moving the legs further apart—to primarily target the glute muscles. Let's break down a banded resistance variation you can do with lunges and squats. You can do this movement as a split squat, where both feet maintain their position, or as a reverse lunge, where the free leg steps backward.

BANDED LATERAL RESISTANCE: LUNGES

1 Starting with the left leg forward, place the band on the inside of your lower left thigh to increase activation of the left adductor.

2 Repeat steps 2 to 6 from the split squat with internal and external rotation on page 79.

3 Maintain the left knee position over the ankle throughout the entire movement. There may be a tendency for the knee to move outward, and you may overcompensate by bringing the knee too far inward.

4 Next, progress to a lunge by placing the right leg forward, placing the band on the outside of the lower right thigh.

5 Repeat step 2.

6 Maintain the right knee position over the ankle throughout the entire movement. There may be a tendency for the knee to move inward, or you may overcompensate by moving the knee too far outward.

If you find that the asymmetrical stance is painful, even with pelvic rotation, modifying to an even stance squat with banded resistance can still strengthen asymmetrically.

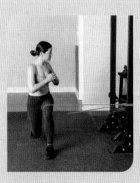 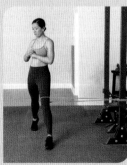 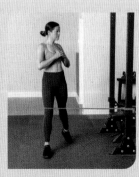 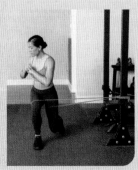

SINGLE-LEG MOVEMENTS: MODIFICATION STRATEGIES

Single-leg exercises, such as the split squat or lunge, can become challenging in the second trimester, especially if you are suffering from pelvic girdle pain. If you're experiencing this, try the modification strategies below to find a variation that allows you to continue training one leg at a time without pain.

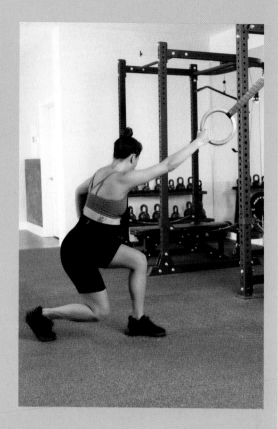

- **Decrease weight shifting:** This can include modifying your lunge from alternating each leg to only doing one leg at a time. This decreases the stabilization demand.

- **Decrease overall movement:** To modify a walking lunge, where both feet are moving, switch to a reverse lunge, where only one foot is moving. You can go even further and switch from a reverse lunge to a split stance, where no feet are moving.

- **Even the stance:** If an asymmetrical stance continues to be painful, you can switch from a lunge position to a squat.

You can also try adding support to your lunges or squats by holding onto rings or a supportive surface. This helps decrease the amount of weight your lower body is supporting, which alleviates some of the stabilization demands.

Modifications to Single-Leg Movements

STANDARD	MODIFICATION, LEVEL 1	MODIFICATION, LEVEL 2	MODIFICATION, LEVEL 3
Two legs moving	One leg moving	Stationary	Even stance
Walking lunges	Reverse lunge	Split squat	Squat

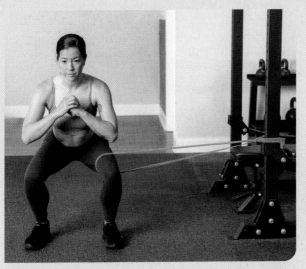
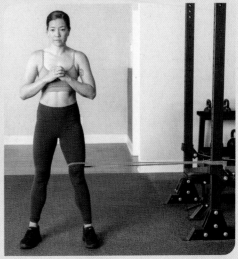

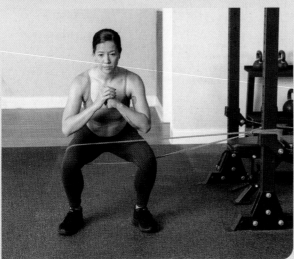
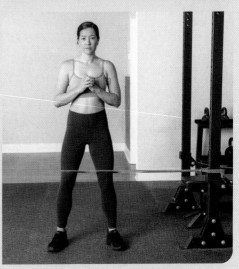

BANDED LATERAL RESISTANCE: SQUATS

1 Starting with the left side, step the left leg into the band so it is resting on the inner left thigh.

2 Inhale to lower to the bottom of the squat.

3 Exhale to stand up.

4 Maintain the left knee position over the ankle the entire movement. There may be a tendency for the knee to move outward, and you may overcompensate by bringing the knee too far inward.

5 Then progress to the right side. Step both legs into the band, so the band is resting on the outside of the right thigh.

6 Repeat steps 2 to 3.

7 Maintain the right knee position over the ankle the entire movement. There may be a tendency for the knee to move inward, or you may overcompensate by moving the knee too far outward.

BULGARIAN SPLIT SQUAT

This exercise strengthens the quads and glutes. Keep in mind that typically the right-side quad and glute are weaker than the left side. Because of this, you have the option to perform this exercise solely on the right side or opt for more repetitions on the right side as compared to the left, such as 5 repetitions on the left side and 10 repetitions on the right.

You can also incorporate hip rotation to further strengthen the glute and increase hip mobility. If you're having pelvic pain, you may observe that increasing internal rotation at the hip decreases or alleviates pelvic pain. This is due to strengthening of the glute muscles, a shift in pelvic floor tension, and improved alignment of the pelvic joints, which aids in stabilization.

1 Start in the elevated split squat position, with your right foot on the floor and left foot elevated behind you. This will target the right glute and quad.

2 Inhale to lower to the bottom of the split squat position. As you lower, rotate the pelvis toward the right upper thigh. You should feel more of a stretch in the right glute and hamstring. Maintain weight in the big toe and keep the right knee stacked over the ankle.

3 Exhale to stand back up to the starting position. As you stand up, rotate to find an open hip position.

4 Repeat for 10 repetitions.

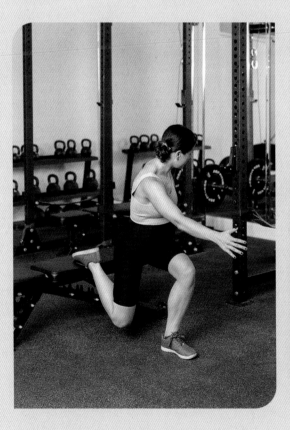

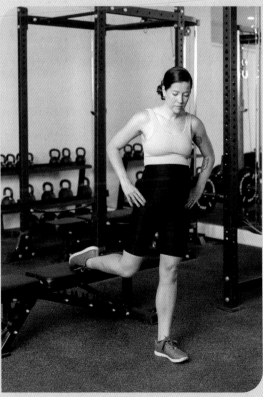

COPENHAGEN PLANK

This exercise strengthens the adductor and the inner thigh muscles. Remember that the left side adductor tends to be weaker than the right, so you can perform this exercise exclusively on the left side or opt for an extended duration on the left side compared to the right. For instance, you might hold the position for 30 seconds on the left side and only 15 seconds on the right side. If this position feels unattainable, try the side-lying hip abduction with ball squeeze on page 56.

1 Begin on your side with your right forearm on the floor, with your elbow stacked under your shoulder.

2 Place your left leg on an elevated surface, such as a bench or couch, and the right knee on the floor. The higher you place your leg on the surface, the easier it will be. For example, the knee will be easier than the ankle. If you do not have an elevated surface, choose the floor Copenhagen plank modification.

3 Place weight into your left leg as you lift your hips and right leg off the floor. If you need an easier modification, keep the right knee on the floor for additional support.

4 Maintain this position for 10 to 30 seconds.

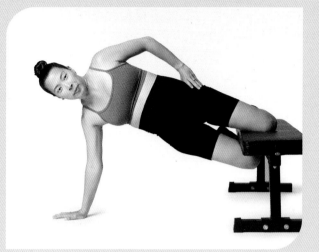
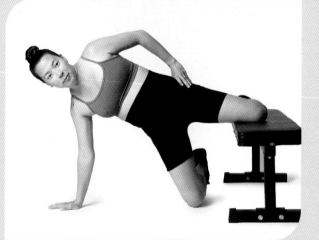
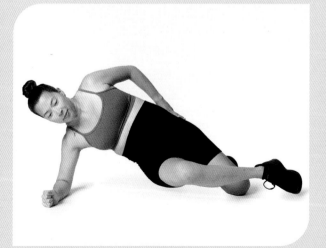

LONG-BANDED ALL-FOURS FIRE HYDRANT

This exercise can also strengthen the gluteus medius and adductor, but in a more supportive position, which you may find easier if you have a lot of pelvic pain. In this variation, you use a long resistance band similar to the squat and lunge with banded resistance (see page 88), with the left leg emphasizing adduction and the right leg emphasizing abduction.

1 Start in a tabletop position with your knees wide, and with your left side toward the point of attachment.

2 Place the left leg into the band so the band is in contact with the inside of your left thigh.

3 Exhale to pull the left knee toward the right knee. You should feel the left inner thigh turn on.

4 Inhale to return to the starting position. Repeat for 10 to 20 repetitions.

5 Switch to the right side by maintaining your body orientation with the left side toward the point of attachment, and place both legs into the band so the band is in contact with the outside of the right leg.

6 Start with both knees closer to each other.

7 Exhale to push the right leg outward. You should feel the right glute turn on more.

8 Inhale to return to the starting position. Repeat for 10 to 20 repetitions.

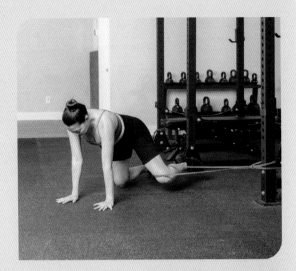

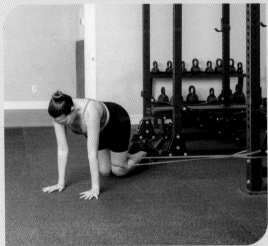

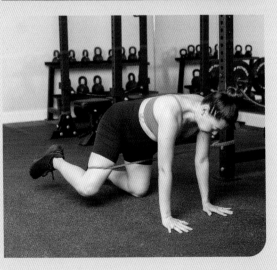

QUICK REFERENCE CHART FOR PELVIC ASYMMETRY EXERCISES

ISSUE	SOLUTION	EXERCISES
Left side: Pelvis sits more forward • Externally rotated • Abduction • Anterior pelvic tilt	Tighter and needs mobility: • Hip flexors and quads • Lats	• Hip flexor and quad release • Forward-leaning lat release • Standing lat release
Bilateral external rotation with arched back* • External rotation • Abduction • Anterior pelvic tilt	Longer and needs strengthening: • Hamstring • Adductor	• Deadlifts • Copenhagen planks
Right side: Pelvis sits more backward • Internally rotated • Adduction • Posterior pelvic tilt	Tighter and needs mobility: • Hamstring and adductor Longer and needs strengthening: • Glute and quadricep	• Adductor rock back • Bulgarian split squats

*If you favor this bilateral position, you will want to focus on this for both sides.

BIOMECHANICAL PATTERNS

The second common cause of pelvic girdle pain relates to biomechanical patterns, which involve how you move your body. When you move, the muscles should cause force closure on the pelvic joints. Force closure involves the supportive structures coming together to stabilize the joint during movement, decreasing unnecessary movement at the joint. If the supporting muscles hinder force closure, it can lead to excessive joint movement, potentially causing discomfort or instability. It doesn't mean your pelvic joints are inherently unstable, but your body might react by tensing up to compensate for perceived instability. This tension alters movement patterns, limiting overall mobility, which is often problematic during pregnancy.

Biomechanical patterns involve the synchronized movement of myofascial slings. These slings consist of interconnected muscles and surrounding fascia, collaborating to offer stability and transmit forces during body movements. They create functional chains spanning various body regions, which are crucial for balance, movement coordination, and postural support.

The myofascial slings supporting the pelvic girdle include the anterior oblique sling, posterior oblique sling, lateral sling, and deep longitudinal sling. These interconnected systems play a key role in supporting and stabilizing the pelvic area. Let's explore each sling with exercises you can incorporate into your workout routine that both support core strengthening and pelvic stability.

Anterior Oblique Sling

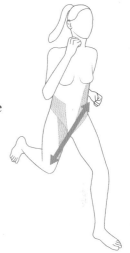

Starting on the front side of the body, you have the anterior oblique sling that forms an X from the chest to the inner thigh muscles on the opposite side. These slings intersect at the pubic symphysis, the front pelvic joint. They support rotational movements like torso twists and help stabilize the pelvis during activities such as walking and lunging.

To strengthen and enhance the functionality of the anterior oblique sling, both ends of the sling need to contract simultaneously. This often involves front rotational movements, where the shoulder and opposite knee move toward the body's center. The following exercise targets the anterior oblique sling.

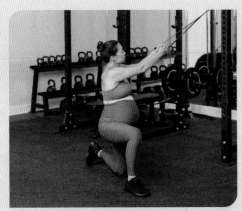

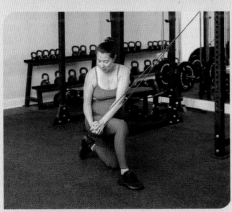

DIAGONAL BANDED PULL-DOWN

This exercise can be done seated, half kneeling, split squat, or standing; you can maintain a stationary position with your legs; or you can incorporate movement with a split squat.

1 Attach a band above eye level to a sturdy structure or over the top of your door frame.

2 Reach toward the point of attachment with tension still in the band.

3 Exhale to rotate and pull the band down toward the outside knee.

4 Inhale to slowly release tension as you reach back toward the point of attachment.

5 Advance this movement by incorporating a split squat, where you start with both legs extended, then exhale to lower to the bottom of the split squat.

6 Repeat 10 times per side.

Posterior Oblique Sling

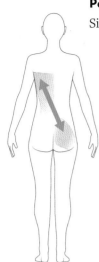

Similar to the anterior oblique sling, the posterior oblique sling forms an X on the back of the body, running from the latissimus dorsi muscle to the opposite gluteal muscle. The intersection of this sling is above the sacroiliac joints. This sling's ends are connected by a strong band of connective tissue that spans the lower back and contributes to the transfer of forces between the upper and lower body. The posterior oblique sling helps stabilize the pelvis during activities like walking and running. Activating the posterior oblique sling involves simultaneously contracting the opposite ends of the sling: the lats with the opposite glute. This can be accomplished with movements that emphasize hip extension and rowing, such as the squat row or lunge row.

SQUAT WITH BANDED ROW

The squat is a more symmetrical position for your pelvis, which may alleviate pelvic pain if single-leg or asymmetrical movements are problematic for you. You can incorporate a banded row to strengthen the posterior oblique sling with any hip extension focused exercise, such as single-leg deadlifts, staggered stance Romanian deadlifts (RDLs), step-ups, and lunges. You can also modify the exercise by squatting to a box, if you need additional support, and you can place a mini band around the thighs for more gluteal activation.

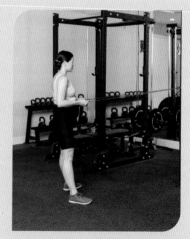

1 Start in a squat position, holding onto a resistance band with both hands.

2 Inhale to lower to the bottom of the squat as you reach forward with the band. This will lengthen the lats and the gluteal muscles.

3 Exhale to stand up as you extend your hips and row the band back.

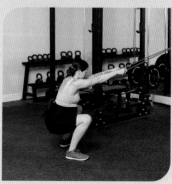

4 If you are feeling any strain in the lower back, tuck the butt underneath at the top of the movement.

5 Repeat 10 times.

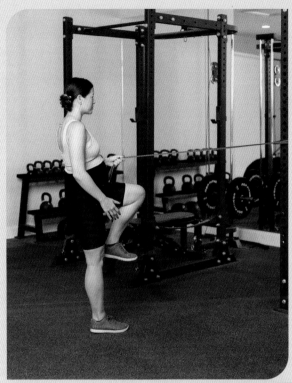

LUNGE WITH BANDED ROW

The lunge offers more stability challenge with the asymmetrical and single-leg stance.

1 Start in a standing or split squat position, holding onto a resistance band with the hand opposite of the working leg (the leg that stays forward).

2 Inhale to lower to the bottom of the lunge, as you reach forward with band. This will lengthen the lats and the gluteal muscles.

3 As you lower to the bottom of the lunge, find internal rotation by rotating the belly to the thigh. Maintain the knee's position over the ankle and keep weight in the big toe of the forward leg.

4 Exhale to stand up as you row the band back. If you are doing a split squat variation, externally rotate at the top by moving the belly away from the forward leg.

5 Repeat 10 times per side.

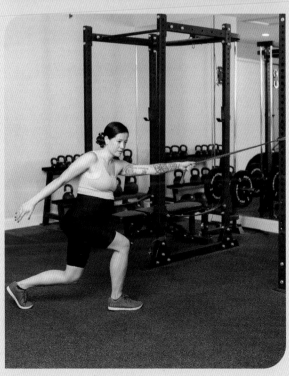

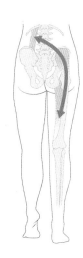

Lateral Sling

The lateral sling starts in the lower back and crosses the opposite leg's gluteus medius and adductor muscles. This sling supports lateral movements, such as stepping sideways. This sling stabilizes the pelvis when you balance on one leg. Exercises that target the lateral sling involve single-leg exercises such as step ups (below) and the lateral band walk (pages 91-92).

STEP-UP WITH BANDED ROW

Step-ups with a banded row are a combination of posterior oblique sling and lateral sling exercises. Step-ups require single-leg stability, and the banded row with hip extension emphasizes stabilization of the sacroiliac joint.

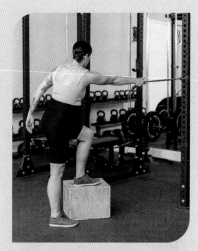

1 Starting with one foot elevated on a box or step-up surface, grab the band with the opposite hand of the elevated foot. A helpful hint is to focus on opposite sides working together.

2 At the bottom of the movement, find internal rotation by rotating the belly to the thigh. Maintain weight in the big toe and alignment of the knee over the ankle.

3 Then reach forward with the band to find length in both the glute and the lats.

4 Exhale to step up on top of your box or step-up surface, as you row the band back.

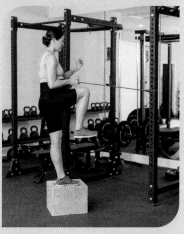

5 If you feel any strain in your low back at the top, focus on tucking the butt underneath at the top.

6 Inhale to lower back down, finding internal rotation at the hip as you reach forward with the band.

7 Repeat 10 times per side.

LATERAL BAND WALK MODIFICATIONS

This exercise strengthens the outer glute muscles and supports single-leg stability. However, this exercise can be problematic if abduction, or spreading the legs, is painful. The following lists modifications for the lateral band walk, regressing toward a more accessible variation if you find abduction painful.

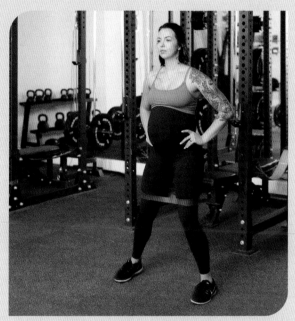

Variation 1:
Lateral Band Walk

1 Place a mini or glute band around your legs. The higher the band, the easier the movement. Place it around the knee, ankles, or even arches of your feet.

2 Place weight in your trail leg.

3 Hover the lead leg momentarily to balance on the trail leg.

4 Then drive through the trail leg to spread the legs apart.

5 Place the lead foot back on the floor and bring the feet together and repeat for 20 to 30 steps. Then switch directions.

If you have space limitations, you can alternate directions for your steps, such as two steps right, then two steps left.

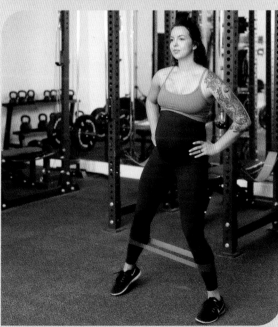

LATERAL BAND WALK MODIFICATIONS, CONT.

Variation 2:
All-Fours Fire Hydrant

If you find the lateral band walk is painful, increasing your base of support from one point of contact to three can alleviate your pain.

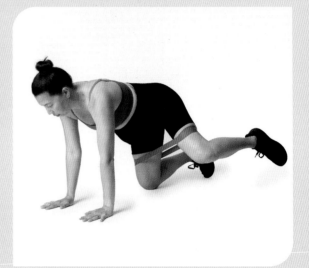

1 Start in a tabletop position. Place a mini band around the thighs.

2 Hover one knee off the floor.

3 Exhale to push the knee out.

4 Inhale to bring the knees back together.

5 Repeat for 10 to 20 repetitions per side.

Variation 3:
Clam Shells

If the tabletop position is still painful, regressing to a side-lying position can take the weight out of the legs to decrease pelvic pain.

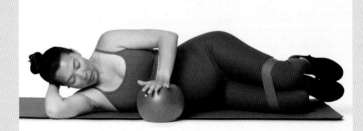

1 In a side-lying position, place a mini band around your thighs.

2 Stack your hips on top of one another and maintain this position as you spread the knees apart. Option to place your hips to a wall to prevent any rocking backward.

3 Exhale to spread the knees apart.

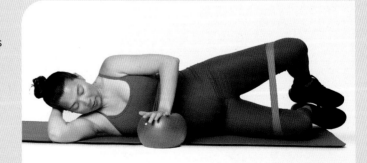

4 Inhale to bring the knees back together and repeat 10 to 20 times.

5 Then you can progress to having the band around the ankles to find internal rotation. Exhale to spread the ankles apart; inhale to bring them back together.

6 Repeat 10 to 20 times.

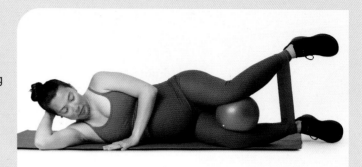

Variation 4: Hip Thrust with Isometric Banded Abduction

If any abduction is painful, opt for a hip thrust with a band activation of the outer glutes without any actual movement to alleviate pain.

1 In a hip thrust position, with your back on an elevated surface such as a bench or your couch, place a mini band around your thighs.

2 Step the feet wide enough to where you are resisting adduction from the mini band. Maintain this tension for the duration of the movement.

3 Exhale to extend in the hips.

4 Inhale to lower the hips back down.

5 Repeat 10 to 20 times.

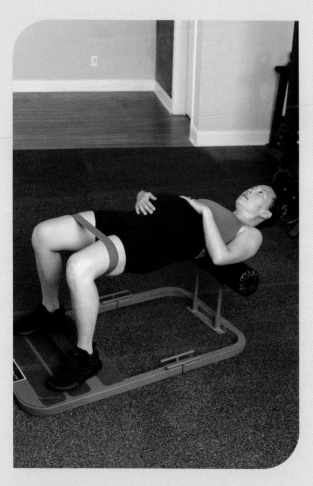

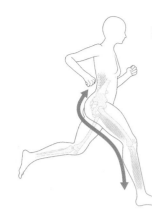

Deep Longitudinal Sling

The deep longitudinal sling involves muscles running along the back of the body, including the erector spinae muscles, which help extend the spine and the hamstrings. This sling supports activities like walking and running by transmitting forces from the lower body through the back to the upper body, contributing to a coordinated and efficient gait. To target the deep longitudinal sling, we use hinge-focused exercises, such as suitcase deadlifts.

SUITCASE DEADLIFTS

The suitcase deadlift is a hinge exercise that targets the deep longitudinal sling and uses only resistance on one side. Because of the one-sided loading, you will also need to resist rotation in your torso toward the side where you are holding the weight. You can use either a long resistance band, a weight, or a combination of both. The resistance band will provide variable resistance, which means it changes in difficulty throughout the movement. The bottom of the movement will be easier than the top of the movement where the band is more stretched. Weights provide nonvariable resistance, which means the difficulty is the same throughout the movement.

1 Hold one weight or band in one hand.

2 Inhale to hinge the hips back as you maintain your torso position.

3 Exhale to stand back up. Repeat 10 times per side.

4 Increase the challenge by holding a band in one hand and a weight in the other.

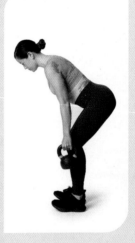
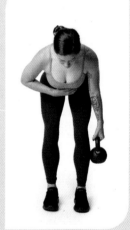
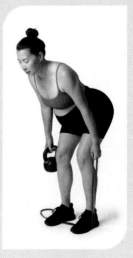
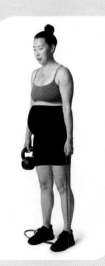

SAMPLE PELVIC STABILITY WORKOUT

Use the following workout template as a guide for a pelvic stability workout or develop your own using the exercises listed throughout this chapter.

LEVEL	EXERCISES		
Warm-up	SPD reset with ball squeeze SJD reset with all-fours hip shift		
Easy	A: 2 rounds 8x squat with lateral resistance (per side) 8x all-fours fire hydrant (per side)	B: 2 rounds 5x seated diagonal pull-down (per side) 5x suitcase deadlift with band (per side)	C: 2 rounds 5x step up with banded row (per side) 5x hip thrust with banded resistance
Moderate	A: 2 rounds 8x split squat with lateral resistance (per side) 15 seconds Copenhagen plank with right knee down (left side)	B: 3 rounds 5x half-kneeling diagonal pull-down (per side) 5x suitcase deadlift with weight (per side)	C: 3 rounds 8x step up with banded row (per side) 8x lateral band walk (per direction)
Advanced	A: 3 rounds: 8x Bulgarian split squat (right side) 30 seconds Copenhagen plank (left side)	B: 3 rounds: 5x split squat diagonal pull-down (per side) 5x suitcase deadlift with weight and band (per side)	C: 3 rounds: 8x step up with banded row and weight (per side) 8x lateral band walk (per direction)

KEY TAKEAWAYS

In the second trimester, you'll begin to modify your lifts to accommodate your belly and to increase comfort in your movements. If you experience any pelvic girdle pain, know that there is hope and you can find relief during your pregnancy. Let's advance to the final trimester and explore modifications during those last months.

SIX
THE THIRD TRIMESTER

AS YOU TRANSITION INTO THE THIRD TRIMESTER, there will be daily fluctuations in how you feel: Some days, you may be more energized, and others, you may want to just lie on the couch and nap. You can exercise and move your body, even with fatigue! But the intensity level of that exercise should decrease to accommodate your energy levels.

As pregnancy progresses, you may find that the more days you take off from your workouts, the more pain you wind up experiencing. Continuing your workout routine until birth can help you stay comfortable and pain-free. Of course, you'll need to continue modifying your exercises from the second trimester to accommodate your growing belly. Don't let it affect your ego! Preparing for birth (and parenthood!) involves letting go of your expectations so you can be open to the experience as it really is.

THIRD-TRIMESTER LIFTING MODIFICATIONS

In the third trimester, you will likely need to modify most of your main lifts. Some movements, such as squats, may look the most similar to prepregnancy, but other movements, like pull-ups or hip thrusts, may look completely different. Modifications are mainly due to your growing belly, shifts in your center of gravity, postural tendencies, and discomforts as you get closer to your due date. Common ways to modify exercise in the third trimester include:

- Increasing support in your movements
- Decreasing the range of motion
- Adjusting the setup

These modifications will vary from exercise to exercise. Still, the overall goal is the same: to make the movement more accessible and comfortable as you maintain your fitness through the entirety of your pregnancy.

INCREASING SUPPORT IN MOVEMENTS

As you move into the third trimester, there are a number of musculoskeletal changes that occur in response to the change in the distribution of weight in your body. There is an increased curvature of the lower spine (known as *lumbar lordosis*), your center of gravity has shifted dramatically forward and upward, and joint laxity, or the movement happening in your joints, will be at its peak. All of these changes can make it harder to stabilize during exercise.

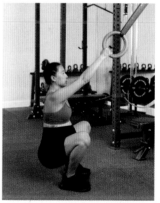

When you increase physical support in your exercises, you can decrease the stabilization demands and make it easier to maintain optimal form to reduce discomfort. For example, you can hold onto a sturdy structure or modify to a more supportive setup, such as a seated position.

Hold onto Rings or a Doorframe

One way to add support for squats or lower body strengthening exercises is by holding onto rings or a sturdy structure, such as a doorframe. This modification can adjust the way you need to balance, and can increase your range of motion.

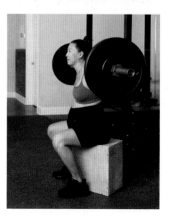

Use a Box

Another squat modification that increases support at the bottom of the lift is the box squat. If you have lower back discomfort with squats, particularly near the bottom of your lift, adding a box can increase your comfort because it increases the support at the bottom of the movement.

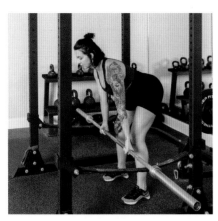

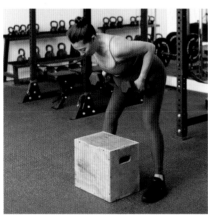

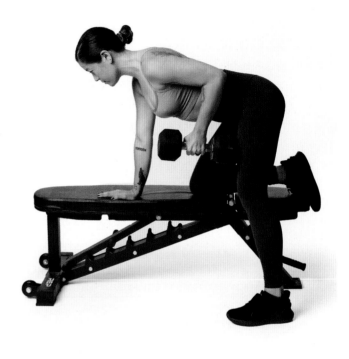

Lower Weights to Safety Straps or Box

Additionally, you can add support at the bottom of upper body exercises, such as the bent-over row, by lowering the barbell to safety straps or the dumbbells to a box. This modification can decrease the strain in your lower back.

Change from Standing to a Seated Position

Upper body modifications to increase support can include changing from a standing position, which requires more joints to stabilize, to a seated position, where there are fewer stabilization demands on the lower body. The upper body's movement is still the same with a standing and seated overhead press, so the same intent and overall movement goal is still being achieved, but in a more supported position.

Increase Points of Contact

Another modification includes increasing the points of contact, or the number of body parts touching a supportive surface. For example, you can modify a bent-over row (only your two feet provide support against the floor) to a single-arm dumbbell row with one hand and knee on the bench and one foot on the floor (increasing to three points of contact).

Decrease Clenching

When you feel stable, you don't clench! Clenching in the pelvic floor is a typical compensation pattern when you feel unstable. This clenching is an attempt to counter the feeling of instability. However, an overly clenched or tense pelvic floor can exacerbate discomfort during your pregnancy, cause issues during labor, and increase pelvic floor concerns postpartum. An overactive pelvic floor can also cause chronic pelvic pain! Therefore, it's important to feel stable in your movements as you exercise to minimize clenching.

DECREASING RANGE OF MOTION

In the third trimester, reducing the overall range of motion with your lifts can be more comfortable, particularly at the end ranges (usually the bottom portion of the exercise). If you feel restriction or discomfort at the bottom of a lift, decreasing the range of motion can increase comfort.

Elevate the Bar or Use a Box

Common ways to decrease range of motion include elevating the bar for the deadlift and the hip thrust. Additionally, you can use a box that is higher than knee level to decrease the range of motion in a squat.

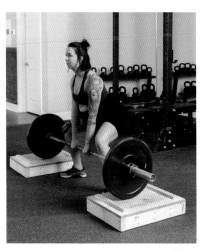

Place Support Alongside Your Pelvis

To decrease range of motion but also increase comfort in the hip thrust, add Fat Gripz or rolled-up hand towels at the edges of your pelvis. These add more space between the bar and your belly, increasing your comfort during the lift.

Maintain Optimal Form

If your belly impedes hip flexion, or how much you can bend at your hip, you will tend to round the lower back to perform a deep squat or reach the bottom of a deadlift. It's important to maintain optimal form during your lifts, or you risk injury. If you need to decrease your range of motion to do that, you absolutely should!

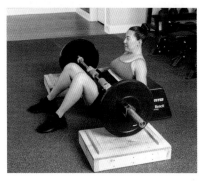

ADJUSTING THE SETUP

In the third trimester, certain positions can feel uncomfortable. Adjusting your position can make the exercise much more comfortable.

Switch from a Supine to an Upright or Inclined Position

A supine or belly-down position can be very uncomfortable. Adjusting your setup to a seated or inclined position can make the exercise much easier. For example, you can modify from a flat bench press to an incline dumbbell press or standing chest press.

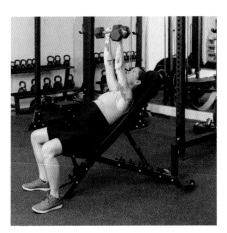 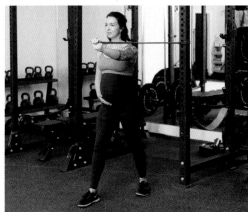

Switch from a Horizontal to a Kneeling Position

The hip thrust can be modified from a horizontal setup to a vertical set up by adjusting to a kneeling variation with either a resistance band or cable machine. The kneeling position can feel more accessible than a horizontal position, and the banded variation may feel more comfortable against your belly as opposed to the barbell.

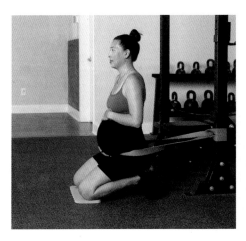 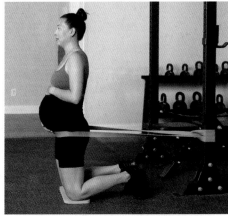

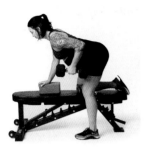 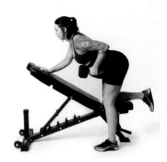 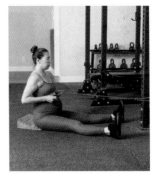

Use a Yoga Block for Stability

In a bent-over or single-arm row where the belly is toward the floor, you can rest your hand against a yoga block or an incline bench to adjust to a more upright position. A seated row is another option.

Switch to Free Weights

You may want to switch from using barbells and heavier weights to free weights, such as dumbbells or kettlebells. The setup for free weights and bands tends to be more accessible, which may be helpful when you are easily fatigued during the last stage of pregnancy. Being mentally okay with letting go of the barbell can also be a part of birth preparation!

Switch to Resistance Bands

Resistance bands are even more accessible than heavy free weights. For example, you can modify the hip thrust to a banded variation in a horizontal position.

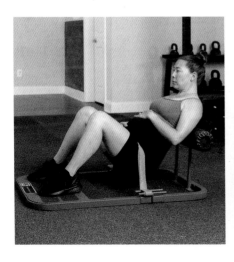 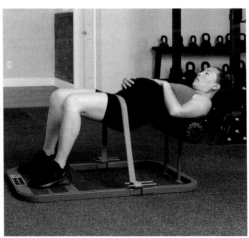

COMMON THIRD-TRIMESTER MOVEMENT MODIFICATIONS

MOVEMENT	MODIFICATION
Squats	Box squats
	Supported squats
Deadlift (hinge)	Sumo deadlift
	Elevated sumo deadlift
	Kettlebell deadlift
	Banded good mornings
Hip thrust	Elevated hip thrust
	Banded hip thrust
	Unweighted hip thrust or glute bridge
	Kneeling hip thrust (bands or cable)
Lunges (single leg movements)	Walking or reverse lunges
	Split squat
	Squat with unilateral loading (bands or weights)
Bench press (horizontal push)	Bench press
	Floor press
	Incline press (dumbbell or bar)
	Standing incline press (bands or cable)
	Standing chest press (bands or cable)
Rows (horizontal pull)	Supported bent-over row (barbell or dumbbells)
	Single-arm row
	Inclined single-arm row
	Seated row (bands or cable)
	Seated single-arm row (band or cable)
Overhead press (vertical push)	Standing overhead press (barbell or free weights)
	Seated overhead press
	Single-arm overhead press (standing or seated)
	Half-kneeling overhead press with pull-down
	Incline press (dumbbell or bar)
	Standing incline press (bands or cable)
Pull-ups (vertical pull)	Lat pull-down
	Straight-arm pull-down
	Ring rows

SAMPLE THIRD-TRIMESTER WORKOUT

In my experience, resistance training is the best way to maintain comfort during the third trimester and support the opening of the pelvis as you prepare for birth. But that doesn't mean you should avoid aerobic activity, such as going for a walk. Moderate aerobic activity 2 or 3 times a week can still be beneficial as a part of your prenatal workout routine.

Use the following workout template as a guide for your third-trimester workouts or develop your own using the exercises listed throughout this chapter. I break down pelvic opening exercises, the birth prep circuit, and labor preparation workout in chapter 7.

SAMPLE THIRD TRIMESTER WORKOUT

	LOWER BODY WORKOUT	UPPER BODY WORKOUT	PELVIC OPENING-FOCUSED WORKOUT	LABOR PREPARATION WORKOUT
Warm-Up	Supported standing hip shift Breathing drill	All fours hip shift Breathing drill	Birth prep circuit	Birth prep circuit
Workout	**A: 3 rounds** 10x squat 8x lateral step-up (per side) 90/90 side opener **B: 3 rounds** 10x deadlift 8x staggered stance RDL with banded row per side Back expansion Breathing drill **C: 2 to 3 rounds** 6x Bulgarian split squat (per side) 10x side lying hip abduction per side 10x bird dog with dumbbell row (per side)	**A: 3 rounds** 10x bench press 8x Pallof press with rotation (per side) 10x farmer carry Standing marches per side **B: 3 rounds** 10x bent-over row 10x diagonal banded pull-down per side Seated thoracic mobility **C: 2 to 3 rounds** 8x floor press and knee press (per side) 10x seated row Seated hip circles	**A: 3 rounds** 8x squat 10x adductor rock back per side Deep squat opener mobility **B: 3 rounds** 8x reverse lunge and row with IR bias 10x single leg curl per side Standing hip shift with lean **C: 2 to 3 rounds** 10x straight leg deadlift with banded pull-down 5x hip airplanes per side 5x squat roll back with IR bias	**5 rounds:** 15 seconds kettlebell swings Birth ball–focused labor positions

COMMON THIRD-TRIMESTER CONCERNS

In the third trimester, you are likely dealing with more of the common discomforts of pregnancy. I firmly believe that pain is not a requirement of pregnancy. Still, it is reasonable to expect to be uncomfortable at some point. Common issues you could encounter during the third trimester include tailbone pain, lower back pain, rib pain, and sleep issues. Let's explore how these four common issues in the third trimester can be resolved with movement.

TAILBONE PAIN

Tailbone pain is a common discomfort in the last trimester of pregnancy. The tail-bone, technically referred to as the *coccyx*, is a mobile bone that attaches to the sacrum with the sacrococcygeal joint. All the pelvic floor muscles are linked to the tailbone, and its position is influenced by these muscles. When there's an uneven pull in the pelvic floor muscles, the tailbone may shift toward the shortened side, leading to discomfort or pain. Additionally, a history of a previous fall on the tailbone or birth injury could increase the risk of experiencing tailbone pain and pelvic floor tension.

The key to resolving tailbone pain is to release the tension in the posterior pelvic floor using exercises like the all-fours hip shift (see page 105) or the standing hip shift (see page 125). For more pelvic floor release exercises, see chapter 7.

Other Tailbone Relief Exercises

Exercises described in other chapters may be useful for tailbone pain, including:

BACK EXPANSION BREATHING DRILL (PAGE 114)

Standing hip shift (page 125)
Supported standing hip shift (page 125)
Leaning hip shift (page 125)

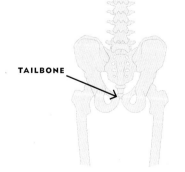

TAILBONE

In addition to movement techniques, you can work with a professional for manual release techniques, either internal or external. A pelvic floor physical therapist or an occupational therapist can support you in manual release techniques during pregnancy, which may require clearance from your medical provider.

If you are suffering from other pelvic floor issues, it is worth connecting with a professional to address your individual concerns, such as constipation, hemorrhoids, vulvar swelling and varicosities, and continence issues.

LOWER BACK PAIN

Lower back pain is a common prenatal issue: More than 60 percent of women complain of lower back pain during pregnancy. Lower back pain can be complex, as the cause may be interpreted differently from person to person. But, if you are experiencing lower back pain, you need to look beyond just the lower back or lumbar spine; the thoracic spine (above the lower back) and the pelvis (below the lower back) need to move well to support the function of the lower back. If there is limited movement in the thoracic spine and pelvis, the lumbar spine often compensates, which could lead to more irritation and pain.

Lower back pain may be due, but not limited, to:

- Limited or restricted thoracic and pelvic movement
- Muscular imbalance
- Muscular strain
- Fatigue
- Sacroiliac joint dysfunction or pelvic girdle pain
- Joint irritation or disc injury

One of the most common reasons for lower back pain is the inability to move your spine to change the position of your rib cage and pelvis. Your spine's mobility affects your posture and breathing strategy. How you position yourself can influence your muscular balance and control, and how you breathe can influence your stability.

During pregnancy, you may find yourself stuck in certain positions for prolonged periods, resulting in muscular fatigue that

ALL-FOURS HIP SHIFT

The all-fours hip shift stretches the back part of your pelvic floor, which releases an uneven pull.

1 Start in a tabletop position.

2 Place a yoga block under one knee.

3 Shift weight toward elevated knee.

4 If needed, use the other leg to push you into the elevated hip by pressing the lower knee into a wall. If usually the opposite leg assists in shifting your weight to the elevated hip, ensure that the opposite knee stays lower than the elevated knee.

5 Round your back.

6 Inhale to expanding in the back. You will feel increased pressure in the back and posterior pelvic floor. If you do not feel a stretch in the posterior pelvic floor, try to round more in your back or shift the weight over more.

7 Exhale to pull the rib cage and pelvis closer together on the front side of the body to find more of a rounded back position.

8 Maintain this position for 5 to 10 breaths.

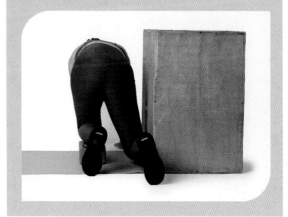

could contribute to lower back pain. Sitting in the same position for lengthy periods can also contribute to lower back pain. Movement is vital to maintaining lower back comfort! Remember, your best posture is the next one—you need to be able to move into different positions without compensating.

Spinal and pelvic mobility exercises, such as thoracic mobility, pelvic tilting, and hip circles, can support your positioning and improve your breathing mechanics. You can incorporate thoracic and pelvic mobility exercises daily or several times a week.

You may have heard that you shouldn't twist or rotate during pregnancy, but this is untrue, as we discussed in chapter 3. Your spine needs to turn as a part of its ordinary and necessary functioning. While you do want to avoid deep abdominal compression twists, thoracic spine rotation is necessary and can help alleviate lower back pain.

The thoracic spine moves in three directions:

- Flexion and extension, or rounding and arching in the spine
- Lateral flexion or extension, or compressing/stretching the side of the body
- Transverse movement, or rotation and twisting

You want to include all three directions when incorporating thoracic mobility into your routine. Here are a few exercises that can help you work on that!

Seated Thoracic Mobility Routine

This routine (page 106) incorporates all three directions of movement of the thoracic spine. These exercises can be done from a seated or kneeling position.

RIB PAIN

Rib pain is another common complaint and can vary in severity and sensation. If you are experiencing right upper abdominal pain that appears to be rib pain, it is important to discuss your symptoms with your provider because it may be related to preeclampsia.

Rib pain not associated with preeclampsia could be related to the function of the diaphragm, the position of the rib cage, and the strain on the attaching musculature. The diaphragm, the primary muscle that supports our breathing, is at the base of the rib cage, separating the thoracic and abdominal cavities. The diaphragm's movement alters the volume of the thoracic cavity, which manages the pressure for the lungs to move air in and out.

During pregnancy, your diaphragm flattens and its range of motion decreases, which could affect rib cage positioning and lead to compression, usually on the right side. This can cause discomfort or pain near the bottom of the rib cage. The solution is to create more space with side-body openers.

SEATED CAT/COWS

The start of the thoracic mobility routine is flexion and extension, or moving the spine front to back. The seated cat/cow movement involves arching the back to feel a stretch in the front of the body, and then rounding the back to feel a stretch in the back of the body. You do not need to find your deepest arch and round—move in a range that feels comfortable, not painful, for you!

1 Start in a seated position.

2 Look up toward the ceiling as you arch in your back, feeling a stretch in the front side of the body.

3 Then look toward the floor as you round in your back, feeling a stretch in the back side of the body.

4 Repeat 5 to 10 times.

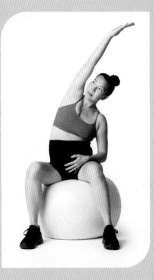

SEATED SIDE OPENER

The next movement in the thoracic mobility routine is lateral movement of the spine. After moving the spine front to back, move it sideways before you progress to rotation.

1 Start in a seated position.

2 Reach one arm overhead.

3 Then stretch that arm toward the opposite side to create a curved position in the side of your body. You should feel a stretch from the hip up toward the arm in the stretched side.

4 To add a mild twist, either rotate the chest more upward or downward to change the sensation in the side of the body.

5 Hold the stretch for 5 to 10 slow breaths or 30 seconds.

SEATED ROTATIONS

Rotation is the third and last step of the sequence and should only be done after warming up the spine in the first two steps.

1 In a seated position, place the hand on the inside of the same side knee (less intense) or outside of the opposite knee (more intense).

2 Use that hand to create leverage to twist the upper body.

3 Rotate 5 to 10 times, then switch sides.

You can also use support devices to find relief from lower back pain, such as using supported seat devices or cushions, belly bands, or support garments. Additionally, you can work with a physical therapist on your postural tendencies and breathing strategies.

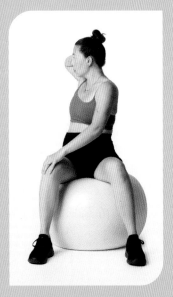

IMPORTANT NOTE ABOUT PREECLAMPSIA

Preeclampsia is a pregnancy complication related to high blood pressure and may also involve some end-organ dysfunction. Right upper abdominal pain, known as *right upper quadrant pain*, and another symptom in the list below, could indicate preeclampsia. If you are experiencing rib pain, it's essential to tell your provider, especially if you have a history of high blood pressure.

Signs and Symptoms of Preeclampsia

- Right upper quadrant pain
- Headache not relieved by remedies/pain relievers
- Changes in vision, such as blurred or spots in vision
- Sudden severe swelling of hands and feet (not diagnostic but a common symptom)
- High blood pressure

RIB CAGE DISCOMFORT RELIEF EXERCISES

Seated side opener	Page 107

Thoracic mobility exercises
- Seated Cat/Cows — Page 107
- Seated Side Opener — Page 107
- Seated Rotations — Page 107

Lat releases
- Forward-leaning lat release — Page 133
- Standing lat release — Page 116

Rib pain can also be associated with overstretching or strain of the abdominal muscles attached to the rib cage. If rib pain is due to overstretching, external support such as a belly band/support garment or abdominal taping by a professional could provide pain relief.

SLEEP ISSUES

Sleep can feel elusive in the third trimester due to pregnancy insomnia, needing to pee more often, or discomfort. Sleep is crucial for your health, but up to 78 percent of pregnant women complain of sleep issues during the third trimester. Poor sleep quality may be associated with an increased risk of prenatal and postpartum depression, as well as adverse pregnancy outcomes.

If you are experiencing pregnancy insomnia, cognitive behavioral therapy with a perinatal mental health specialist may be helpful. Other options, such as prenatal yoga, prenatal massage, and meditation, can also support your sleep throughout pregnancy.

If you're waking up more than twice a night to pee, it could indicate a pelvic floor issue. Working with a pelvic floor physical therapist may be helpful. Pelvic floor physical therapy can also help if you have hip pain or pain shifting your position in bed.

If you are experiencing hip pain, pain while rolling or shifting your position in bed, or even reflux and heartburn, you can first focus on your sleeping position. An easy way to do this is to place a pillow between your knees and ankles to keep the hips in a more neutral position.

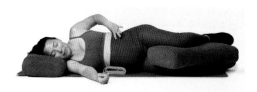

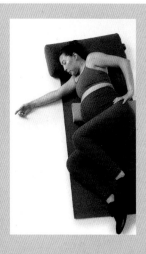

HIP SHIFT WITH PILLOW SQUEEZE

If you are experiencing pain when shifting your position in bed, you can incorporate a hip shift with the pillow squeeze. If you recall from chapter 3, the common postural tendency is left hip forward and right hip backward. This common posture can become more pronounced during pregnancy. Shifting your posture with the left knee moving backward and the right knee moving forward can help bring the pelvis into a more balanced position, making it easier to stabilize.

1 Place a pillow between the knees.

2 Drive the right knee forward.

3 Shift the left hip backward.

4 Squeeze the pillow as you roll or change positions.

5 Roll or change positions.

Another option for changing positions is to come to an all-fours position instead of rolling onto your back. This will be more labor-intensive, but if rolling onto your back from your side is painful, even with a pillow squeeze and hip-shifted position, moving to a tabletop position to switch sides may be the best thing to do.

If you're experiencing pain while rolling or shifting your position in bed, you can squeeze a pillow between your knees as you change position. This squeeze activates the inner thighs, which helps to stabilize the pelvic girdle.

KEY TAKEAWAYS

The final trimester of pregnancy will likely test you as an athlete the most—you will need to modify your exercises and lower overall intensity. And then, add on the common aches and pains that may become more prevalent as you near your due date. But relief is possible and reasonable to achieve, even in this third trimester.

The ability to let go of expectations will only positively serve you as you prepare for birth. Giving birth requires us to surrender and let go of our expectations to open up to this new experience of motherhood. You can mentally prepare for this aspect by learning to surrender to your experience and be willing to let go of certain aspects of your workouts. In the next chapter, we will break down what you can do to physically prepare for birth.

SEVEN
PREPARATION FOR BIRTH

PRENATAL FITNESS PROGRAMS SHOULD BE more than a workout program that excludes sit-ups and crunches while incorporating only "pregnancy-safe" exercises. Prenatal fitness programs should not only guide you through a strong and comfortable pregnancy but also prepare you for birth. In this chapter, we will discuss what you can incorporate into your workout routine to prepare for labor and delivery.

PREPARING FOR BIRTH: OPENING THE PELVIS

In labor, your baby makes their way through your pelvis and pelvic floor. First, they enter the pelvic inlet, twist through the midpelvis, and finally extend their head beneath the pubic arch to crown and be born. We delve deeper into your baby's positions and movements in the pelvis in chapter 8.

Your baby's movement through your pelvis is easier if you can create more space in each pelvic level. The good news is, you don't have to wait until labor to work on this. You can integrate pelvic opening exercises into your prenatal workouts to ensure you've got the movement capacity to make room in your pelvis. Limited mobility in the pelvis can potentially slow down or stall labor.

The pelvis is divided into three levels: the inlet, the midpelvis, and the outlet. In addition, the pelvic floor plays a large role in the midpelvis. Each level responds to different movement patterns. No single movement opens up the entire pelvis. Instead, each level has its unique pattern, expanding the pelvic diameters to create more space for your baby to navigate and rotate.

The joints in the pelvic girdle—the sacroiliac joints, pubic symphysis, and sacrococcygeal joint—play a role in opening these pelvic levels. During pregnancy, these joints experience more significant displacement than when you're not pregnant. This means that movement can significantly influence the pelvis's opening. It's not a rigid set of bones, and the pelvic diameters can expand with movement!

Let's break down how each pelvic level opens and the corresponding exercises you can do during pregnancy to prepare for an easier labor.

THE PELVIC INLET

Starting at the top of the pelvis, we have the pelvic inlet. The inlet is where your baby will first enter or engage into the pelvis. In this section, we break down which movement patterns create more space and the exercises you can include to help open the top of the pelvis.

POSITIONS THAT OPEN THE TOP OF THE PELVIS

BIOMECHANICAL TERM	WHAT IT LOOKS LIKE	HOW IT HELPS
External rotation at the hip	Knees out, ankles in	Creates more space side to side in the pelvic inlet
Abduction at the hip	Wide knees or legs	Creates more space side to side in the pelvic inlet when combined with external rotation
Posterior pelvic tilt	Tucking the butt under Rounding the back Full hip extension	Creates more space front to back in the pelvic inlet by moving the sacral promontory backward
Anterior pelvic tilt	Arched back	Makes external rotation and abduction at the hip easier, which can create more space side to side in the pelvic inlet Changes pubic bone angle, which can make it easier for baby to enter into the pelvis

The top of the pelvis opens more with external rotation and abduction at the hip. External rotation means that the knee rotates outward as the ankle moves inward. Abduction means that the leg is moving away from the center of your body, or a wide knee position. This is a common movement pattern that occurs as you lower to the bottom of a squat. This movement increases the side-to-side diameter of the pelvic inlet and is usually easy to achieve during pregnancy.

Next, the top of the pelvis opens more with a posterior pelvic tilt. A posterior pelvic tilt rotates the sacrum under, which shifts the sacral promontory backward. This creates more space front to back in the pelvic inlet.

There are two scenarios that can support a posterior pelvic tilt. The first is when you fully extend at the hip—picture yourself deadlifting. At the peak of the movement, pushing your hips forward to "lock out" or "complete" the lift can cause the pelvis to tuck under and tilt posteriorly. The second involves having a rounded back, which is more commonly associated with a posterior pelvic tilt. But, if you recall from chapter 3, a posterior pelvic tilt can be more challenging to achieve during pregnancy. As you incorporate pelvic opening exercises, you may want to emphasize being able to achieve a posterior pelvic tilt.

The final movement pattern that creates more space in the top of the pelvis is an anterior pelvic tilt, or arching in the back. An anterior pelvic tilt makes external rotation easier to achieve, so it could enhance the side-to-side opening of the pelvic inlet. Additionally, the arched position can change the pubic bone angle, which can make it easier for your baby to enter the pelvis. This movement pattern also tends to be easy to achieve during pregnancy.

Since both a posterior and an anterior pelvic tilt can increase space, pelvic tilting or front-to-back movement patterns can be helpful when opening the top of the pelvis.

As you prepare to open the pelvic inlet, focus on incorporating exercises that emphasize hip external rotation, mobility and strengthening of the adductors and hamstrings for pelvic mobility, and mobility that makes a posterior pelvic tilt more accessible during pregnancy.

EXERCISES TO OPEN THE PELVIC INLET

Luckily, when it comes to the pelvic inlet, your body tends to naturally lean toward external rotation and hip abduction, along with an anterior pelvic tilt—common postures during pregnancy. This means you often find yourself with a slightly arched or extended spine, and your legs may naturally turn outward.

This position is a big deal in workouts because it's a power position—you can generate a lot of power in your lifts by moving into this position. During pregnancy, most workout programs actually encourage and reinforce this position.

PELVIC INLET OPENING EXERCISES: EXTERNAL ROTATION AND ABDUCTION

STRENGTHENING EXERCISES	MOBILITY EXERCISES
Squats	Deep squat hold
Sumo stance deadlift	Adductor rock back
Hip thrusts	Half-kneeling weighted shifts
Step-ups	Figure Four
Side lunges	Seated 90/90

PELVIC INLET OPENING EXERCISES: POSTERIOR PELVIC TILT (ROUNDING IN THE BACK)

STRENGTHENING EXERCISES	MOBILITY EXERCISES
Deadlifts	Forward-leaning lat release
Staggered-stance deadlifts	Standing lat release
Single-leg deadlifts	Half-kneeling hip flexor release
Poor man's leg curls	Couch stretch

PELVIC INLET OPENING EXERCISES: ANTERIOR PELVIC TILT (ARCHING IN THE BACK)

STRENGTHENING EXERCISES	MOBILITY EXERCISES
Bent-over rows	Hamstring stretches
Single-arm rows	Cat/cows
Bulgarian split squats	
Split squats	

However, as you may notice, the pelvic inlet also requires a posterior pelvic tilt to open, so constantly reinforcing this extended position could ultimately restrict space in the top of the pelvis, making it harder for your baby to enter into the pelvis.

Now, the tricky part might be getting into that rounded posture with your spine and pelvis. In order to overcome this limitation, let's focus on improving the flexibility of your lats, hip flexors, and quadriceps. Strengthening your hamstrings and adductors will also help pull your pelvis into that posterior pelvic tilt position.

In a posterior pelvic tilt, the pelvis is pulled down from the back by the hamstrings and adductors, while the abdominal wall pulls it up from the front. For this to work well, certain muscles need to release or lengthen—namely, the latissimus dorsi, quadriceps, and hip flexor muscles.

The lats often stay shortened during pregnancy due to the common posture of arching the back. This shortening can make it trickier to achieve a posterior pelvic tilt. To release tension in the lats, try exercises like back expansion breathing and lat releases.

SAMPLE PELVIC INLET-OPENING WORKOUT

Here is a sample workout that you can incorporate once a week as a part of your birth preparation. This exercise incorporates movement patterns required to open the top part of the pelvis.

MOBILITY	3 ROUNDS
• 30 seconds of forward lat release (per side) • 30 seconds of hip flexor release with side opener (per side) • 10 repetitions of adductor rock back (per side)	• 10 repetitions of supported squat with pause and rounding at the bottom • 10 repetitions of banded good morning • 10 repetitions of seated pelvic tilts

BACK EXPANSION BREATHING DRILL: ALL-FOURS POSITION

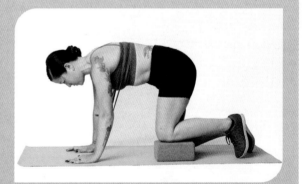

This exercise releases the lats and decreases compression on the back of the rib cage. This can relieve mid-back pain and improve your ability to find a rounded back position.

1 Place a long band or strap across the back of your rib cage, near your bra strap line. This will provide external feedback to help you emphasize the back expansion.

2 Move into a tabletop position.

3 Press the chest and belly away from the floor to find a rounded back position.

4 Inhale to feel the back expand and stretch.

5 Exhale to pull the front of the rib cage and pelvis toward each other, to move deeper into this rounded position.

6 Repeat for 5 to 10 breaths.

COUCH STRETCH

This exercise releases the muscles on the front side of the thigh, which can improve your hip mobility. You can either use an elevated surface to place the back foot on or reach back and grab the foot with your hand.

1 Begin in a half-kneeling stance with your back foot raised against a wall or on an elevated surface, like a couch or gym bench. If lifting the back foot is too intense, simply reach behind and grab your foot to stretch the quad.

2 Tuck the butt underneath to intensify the stretch in the front of the leg.

3 Maintain this tucked position as you slowly sit back toward the elevated foot.

4 Hold this stretch for 5 to 10 breaths, then switch sides.

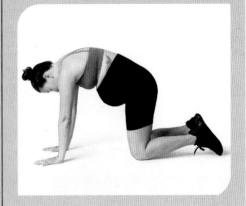

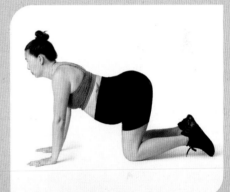

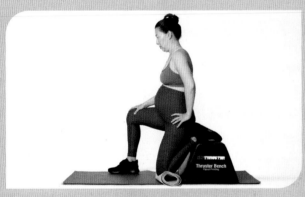

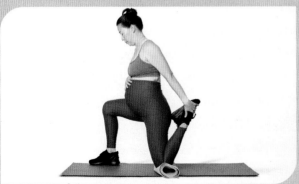

PELVIC TILTS

Pelvic tilts are another great inlet opening exercise that you can incorporate into your prenatal routine (and is a great labor position too). This exercise combines both an anterior pelvic tilt by arching your back and a posterior pelvic tilt by rounding your back. You can do pelvic tilts from a variety of positions, such as seated on a birth ball or chair, on all fours, kneeling, deep squats, and even standing.

STANDING LAT RELEASE

This exercise releases the lats and side of the body. This can relieve tension in the back to improve your ability to find a rounded back position, which will improve your ability to open the pelvis during birth. Additionally, releasing the lats can improve your positioning during prenatal workouts.

1 Standing perpendicular to a door frame or sturdy structure, move in a staggered stance position, with the outside foot backward, and the inside foot forward.

2 Reach overhead to grab the door frame with the outside arm.

3 Allow the hips to shift away from the door frame as you form a curve with your body. You can use your inside arm to push away from the door frame.

4 Hold this position for 5 to 10 breaths, then switch sides.

Moving to the front of your legs, you have the quadriceps and hip flexors. They work together to pull your pelvis downward toward the front of your body. If these muscles are consistently shortened, it might make it challenging for your pelvis to achieve a posterior pelvic tilt. Try incorporating mobility exercises like the couch stretch and hip flexor release to make it easier for you to find that posterior pelvic tilt.

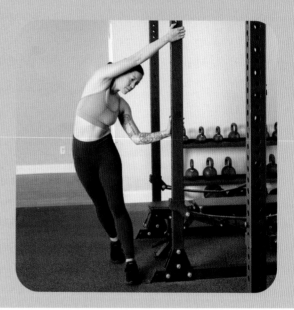

THE MIDPELVIS: THE PELVIC CAVITY

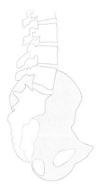

The midpelvis is the bony structure of the pelvis and surrounding pelvic musculature that the baby rotates through during labor. Your baby's main goal in the midpelvis is to rotate through the pelvis.

Movement patterns that create more space in the midpelvis involve asymmetrical or unilateral-type movement patterns, such as side lunges or swaying in the hips, where you shift weight from leg to leg.

The midpelvis has two portions: the upper and the lower midpelvis. Each portion opens opposite the other, so when you open the left upper midpelvis, the right lower midpelvis is also opening.

The upper midpelvis is where the baby begins their rotation into the pelvic cavity. The upper midpelvis opens more with open hip positions, or external rotation and abduction at the hip and an anterior pelvic tilt.

POSITIONS THAT OPEN THE UPPER MIDPELVIS

BIOMECHANICAL TERM	WHAT IT LOOKS LIKE	HOW IT HELPS
External rotation and abduction at the hip	Open hip positions	Creates more space diagonally in the upper half of the pelvis
Anterior pelvic tilt	Arched back	Makes external rotation and abduction at the hip easier, which can create more space diagonally Changes pubic bone angle on this front half, which can make it easier for your baby to begin their rotation into the pelvis

In contrast, the lower midpelvis is where the baby finishes their rotation under the pubic bone. The lower midpelvis opens more in closed hip positions, or with internal rotation and adduction at the hip and a posterior pelvic tilt.

You can understand the difference between an open and closed hip position by considering the relationship between the pelvis and the thigh. If the thigh is moving away from the pelvis, this is an open hip position. If the thigh is moving toward the pelvis, this is a closed hip position.

Although there are two portions to the midpelvis, you can just focus on opening the entire midpelvis by swaying and shifting weight from leg to leg. If you are experiencing an issue during labor, then you want to focus on a specific part of the midpelvis. This may include focusing more on the upper midpelvis if your baby is having trouble engaging into the pelvis, or on the lower midpelvis if your baby is having

POSITIONS THAT OPEN THE LOWER MIDPELVIS

BIOMECHANICAL TERM	WHAT IT LOOKS LIKE	HOW IT HELPS
Internal rotation and adduction at the hip	Closed hip positions Hip shifts	Creates more space diagonally in the lower half of the pelvis. Releases tension in the posterior pelvic floor.
Posterior pelvic tilt	Tucking the butt under Rounded back Full hip extension	Makes internal rotation and adduction easier, which can create more space diagonally Releases tension in the posterior pelvic floor

trouble finishing their rotation under the pubic bone or you have a late labor stall. We discuss labor stalls and solutions in chapter 8.

EXERCISES TO OPEN THE MIDPELVIS

During your prenatal workouts, you can incorporate exercises that ensure you have the movement capability to create space in the midpelvic levels. This includes being able to find both open and closed hip positions, or rotating from external rotation to internal rotation at the hip. You can achieve this with movements like the split squat, where you start in an open hip position, lower to a closed hip position, and then rotate back to an open hip position to finish the movement. This is explained in detail on page 79 in chapter 5.

Similar to the inlet, specific movement patterns can be more challenging to find during pregnancy, such as internal rotation and a posterior pelvic tilt, which are two movement patterns that open the lower midpelvis. As you prepare to open the lower midpelvis for birth, focus on mobility and strengthening exercises that make these movement patterns more accessible.

MIDPELVIS OPENING EXERCISES: UPPER MIDPELVIS (OPEN HIP)

STRENGTHENING EXERCISES	MOBILITY EXERCISES
Cossack lunges	Adductor rock back
Side lunges	Half kneeling weight shifts
Open hip at the top of:	90/90 hip mobility
• Lunges	
• Split squats	
• Staggered-stance RDLs	
• Step-ups	
Lateral band walks	
Fire hydrants	

MIDPELVIS OPENING EXERCISES: LOWER MIDPELVIS (CLOSED HIP)

STRENGTHENING EXERCISES	MOBILITY EXERCISES
Closed hip at the bottom of:	Forward-leaning lat release
• Lunges	Standing lat release
• Split squats	Half-kneeling hip flexor release
• Step ups	Couch stretch
Staggered-stance RDL	Hip shifted breathing drills and pelvic floor releases
Single-leg deadlift	Back expansion breathing drills
Poor man's leg curl	
Deadlifts	

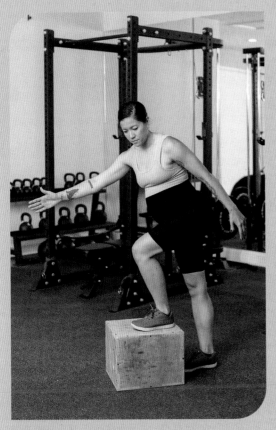

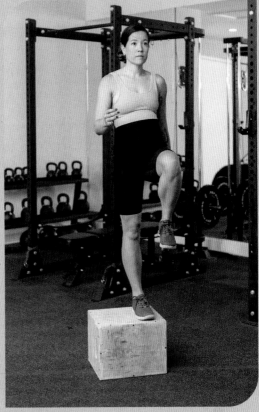

STEP-UPS

Step-ups are a great exercise that emphasizes internal rotation at the bottom and external rotation at the top of the step-up movement. The step-up can be used to prepare to open both the upper and lower midpelvis. You can hold onto weight or incorporate a banded row from page 90.

1 Starting with one foot elevated on a box or step-up surface.

2 At the bottom of the movement, find internal rotation by rotating the belly to the thigh. Maintain weight in the big toe and alignment of the knee over the ankle.

3 Exhale to step up on top of your box or step-up surface to find an open hip position.

4 Inhale to lower back down, finding internal rotation at the hip.

5 Repeat 10 times per side.

There are several variations of the step-up, such as forward, alternating, lateral, and crossover step-ups. Each variation incorporates a different demand, such as changing direction or adjusting glute activation. If pelvic pain is an issue, decrease overall movement, such as keeping your foot on the box the entire time or holding onto a sturdy structure for more support. See chapter 5, page 81, for a modified approach for single-leg movements.

When preparing for birth, you want to focus on ensuring you have the movement capability to open this pelvic level without restriction or limitations. Because most people tend to have an asymmetrical postural tendency, your workouts should not be the same for both sides of your body. This is a hard concept to accept! The upper-left midpelvis tends to be easier to open, while the upper-right midpelvis has more restrictions. Therefore, when working on the upper midpelvis, focus on right-side external rotation, abduction, and an anterior pelvic tilt. Similarly, the lower-right midpelvis tends to be easier to open, while the lower-left midpelvis has more restrictions. Therefore, when working with the lower midpelvis, focus on left-side internal rotation, adduction, and a posterior pelvic tilt.

TIPS FOR INTERNAL ROTATION

Finding internal rotation is an important aspect of improving the function of your hip muscles and glutes and preparing to open the lower pelvis for birth. But internal rotation may be hard to feel in your body! You can use external props, such as a foam roller or resistance bands (see page 80), to increase awareness of what internal rotation should feel like so you can expand this to other movements without the external aids.

You can use a foam roller as a feedback tool to help you feel internal rotation by increasing adduction activation.

1 Place a foam roller between a wall and the inside of your knee.

2 Actively press your knee into the foam roller to feel your inner thigh turn on.

3 Move into an open hip position by rotating your hips toward the wall.

4 Move into a closed hip position by rotating your hips toward the forward leg.

5 As you rotate from an open to closed hip position, pay attention to the sensations that you feel in the supported leg and mimic that sensation in other single leg movements when you are trying to find internal rotation.

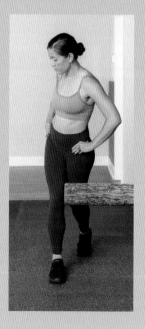
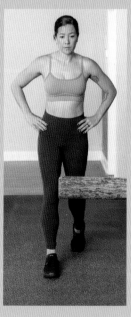

STAGGERED STANCE ROMANIAN DEADLIFT (RDL)

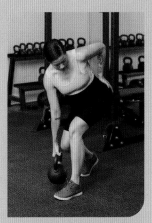

The staggered stance RDL is a unilateral hinge-focused exercise that strengthens the hamstrings and glutes. In the staggered stance RDL, you can focus on finding internal rotation at the bottom and external rotation at the top of the movement. Since this movement is more hinge-focused with increased hamstring activation, it has an increased emphasis on opening the lower midpelvis. You can hold a weight, or do a banded row if you want to emphasize more posterior oblique sling activation.

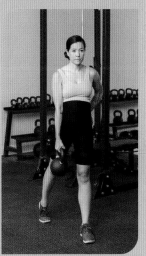

1 Start in a staggered stance position with one foot in front of the other.

2 Hold a weight in the opposite hand of the forward leg.

3 Inhale to lower the weight as you rotate toward the opposite foot.

4 Find internal rotation at the bottom of the movement by rotating the belly to thigh. Keep the front knee stacked over the ankle and weight in the big toe as you lower.

5 Exhale to stand up, as you rotate to an open hip position.

6 Repeat 10 times per side.

SAMPLE PELVIC INLET-OPENING WORKOUT

Here is a sample workout that you could incorporate once a week as a part of your birth preparation. This exercise incorporates movement patterns required to open the middle of the pelvis.

MOBILITY	3 ROUNDS	3 ROUNDS
• 30 seconds per side of adductor rock back • 30 seconds per side of standing hip shift with lean • 30 seconds per side of 90/90 side opener	• 10 repetitions of split squat with left leg banded adduction • 10 repetitions of split squat with right leg banded abduction • 10 repetitions per side of hip shifted pelvic tilts	• 10 repetitions of staggered stance RDL per side • 10 repetitions of lateral step-up with banded row per side

You can still do the same exercise on both sides but adjust the movement with an asymmetrical loading, such as using a resistance band to load the left leg with more adduction emphasis to help with internal rotation and adduction and the right leg with more external rotation and abduction emphasis.

THE PELVIC FLOOR

The pelvic floor is the sling of muscles that sits at the bottom of the pelvic cavity. Incorporating pelvic floor release exercises can affect the opening of the midpelvis.

The pelvic floor can influence your baby's head position during birth. It can support the baby in finding a head flexion or tucking their chin to their chest, which prompts a smaller head circumference. However, if the pelvic floor has uneven tension, it can make the baby's head tilt sideways or cause the baby to extend their head upward or find a deflexed position where they are looking straight forward. Both can cause the baby to appear too large for the pelvis and result in a labor stall or medical interventions during delivery (see more on page 22).

POSITIONS THAT RELEASE THE PELVIC FLOOR

BIOMECHANICAL TERM	WHAT IT LOOKS LIKE	HOW IT HELPS
External rotation and abduction at the hip	Wide knees with ankles closer together, such as deep squats or butterfly pose	Lengthens the front half of the pelvic floor, but shortens the back half of the pelvic floor
Internal rotation and adduction at the hip	Knees closer together with ankles wider, such as hero's pose	Lengthens the back half of the pelvic floor, but shortens the front half of the pelvic floor
Asymmetrical external rotation and internal rotation at the hip	One knee is wide with the ankle closer to the body, and the other knee is closer to the body with the ankle wide, in addition to hip shifts	Lengthens the pelvic floor diagonally from one half of the front pelvic floor to the opposite back pelvic floor

PELVIC FLOOR QUADRANTS

Visualize the pelvic floor in four quadrants: the left and right anterior quadrants and the left and right posterior quadrants. The position of the pelvis influences the tension in these four quadrants.

If you have external rotation in both hips with an anterior pelvic tilt, the front half of the pelvic floor lengthens as the posterior pelvic floor shortens or increases in tension. If you have internal rotation in both hips with a posterior pelvic tilt, the back half of the pelvic floor lengthens as the anterior pelvic floor shortens or increases in tension.

If you favor a right stance, the tailbone shifts to the left as the left posterior quadrant tightens. If you put weight into your left leg, the tailbone shifts in the opposite direction to the right, as the right posterior quadrant tightens. There is no one best position or state of tension for the pelvic floor; rather, you want to ensure that you can shift positions as you move. When you step from foot to foot, the pelvic floor should alternate in rotational tension with each step. However, if you have difficulty moving your pelvic floor out of a specific position, it can affect your baby's position and restrict opening of the lower midpelvis and pelvic outlet.

PELVIC FLOOR RELEASE EXERCISES

During the third trimester, you can prepare for birth by learning to relax the pelvic floor. Deep squats, butterfly pose, and external rotation exercises are often promoted as the *only* exercises for pelvic floor relaxation. However, these movements only stretch the front half of the pelvic floor. They can be incorporated into your pelvic floor mobility routine, but these external rotation–focused exercises overstretch portions of the pelvic floor that are already lengthened, so they should not be the only exercises you do nor dominate your mobility routine.

To release tension in the pelvic floor, incorporate the following exercises:

- Wide-legged positions with the knees out and ankles in, such as deep squats, to release the anterior pelvic floor

- Closed-knee positions with the knees in and ankles out, such as hero pose or supported hinge, to release the posterior pelvic floor

- Combo of open and closed hip positions, such as hip-shifted positions or 90/90, to release rotational tension in the pelvic floor

In all of these pelvic floor release exercises, focus on finding a comfortable position that you can release in and maintain the position for 30 to 60 seconds or 10 full breath cycles.

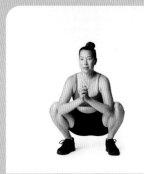
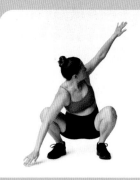

DEEP SQUAT WITH SUPPORT

The deep squat is the traditional pelvic floor release exercise where you are targeting more of the anterior pelvic floor with external rotation at the hip.

1 Start by lowering to the deepest squat you can comfortably find.

2 To further decrease tension in the pelvic floor, at the bottom of the squat, place one hand on the floor and reach upward with the opposite hand to find a twist in the spine.

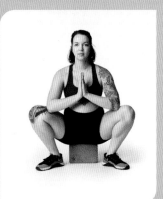
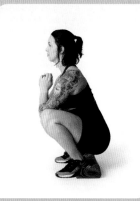

3 If you are having difficulty relaxing at the bottom of the squat, add support, such as sitting on a yoga block or

4 If your heels are lifted off the floor, place a rolled-up towel or yoga mat under your heels for support, as a tippy-toe position can increase tension in the pelvic floor.

90/90 SIDE OPENER

This is an asymmetrical pelvic floor release where one leg is in external rotation in front of you and the other leg is in internal rotation to the side and behind you. You may find that it is easier to have the left leg in front rather than the right leg. If so, spend more time in the more challenging position. Try to sit evenly with both hips. If the bottom position is uncomfortable or inaccessible, sit on a yoga block or small pillow to slightly elevate the hips.

You can also incorporate a side-body stretch by reaching overhead with the arm on the same side as the back leg.

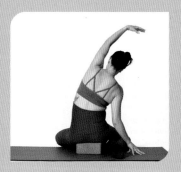
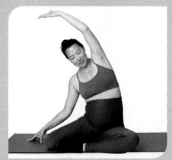

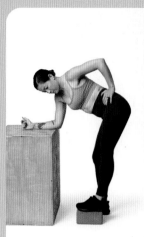

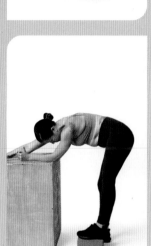

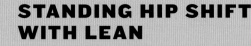

STANDING HIP SHIFT WITH LEAN

The left posterior pelvic floor tends to be in a shortened state. Therefore, finding internal rotation and a posterior pelvic tilt on the left leg tends to be more challenging, and the right-side of the body tends to be more compressed. All three of these movement patterns can be addressed with the standing hip shift with lean, where you prop one leg into internal rotation and stretch the opposite side of the body.

1 Place one foot on an elevated surface roughly 2 to 3 inches (5–8 cm) in height.

2 Hinge the hips back as you place your forearms on an elevated surface roughly hip height or higher.

3 Keep the elevated leg relatively straight as you bend in the support leg.

4 Rotate the belly toward the thigh for internal rotation of the elevated hip. Keep your weight on the big toe of the elevated foot. You should feel more of a stretch in the hamstring and glute.

5 Push the chest away from the floor to round in the back, to incorporate back expansion (thoracic mobility).

6 In the upper body, drag the elbow of the elevated hip side toward the hip to increase the compression on that side of the body and reach across to lengthen the other side of the body.

UNSUPPORTED STANDING HIP SHIFT

You can target the posterior pelvic floor with an unsupported hip shift as well. The same principles apply, but you don't lean onto a supportive surface.

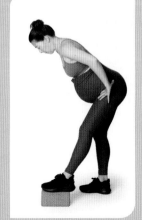

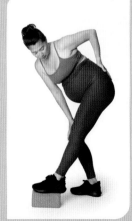

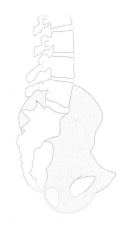

THE PELVIC OUTLET

The pelvic outlet is the bottom of the pelvis, where your baby will finish their rotation under the pubic bone and extend their head under the pubic arch during pushing and crowning.

The bottom of the pelvis opens more with internal rotation and adduction at the hip, or knees in and ankles out. Ensuring you have the capability to achieve both internal rotation and a posterior pelvic tilt is a crucial part of your birth preparation. These movement patterns create more space side to side in the bottom of the pelvis by moving the ischial tuberosities, or sitz bones, further apart.

If you are unsure of where the sitz bones are, sit on your hands to feel for your sitz bones. Start with your knees out and ankles in, and pay attention to where your sitz bones are in your hands. Then rotate your legs so the knees move in and the ankles move out, and feel how your sitz bones move further apart.

Similar to the pelvic inlet, the sacral position influences the opening of the pelvic outlet from front to back. There are two things that can help you create more space: lat activation and not being flat on your back. Lat activation can apply traction to the sacrum to pull the bottom outward, creating more space front to back. Lat activation can also help you achieve a more neutral spine position, which can increase the strength of your pushes. We'll discuss pushing mechanics and strategies in chapter 8 on page 153.

POSITIONS THAT OPEN THE BOTTOM OF THE PELVIS

BIOMECHANICAL TERM	WHAT IT LOOKS LIKE	HOW IT HELPS
Internal rotation and adduction at the hip	Knees in, ankles out	Creates more space side to side in the bottom of the pelvis by moving the sitz bones apart
Posterior pelvic tilt	Tucking the butt under Rounded back Full hip extension	Makes internal rotation and adduction easier, which can create more space diagonally Releases tension in the posterior pelvic floor
Lat engagement	Pulling or rowing with palms up Elbows into side	Creates traction to pull the bottom of the sacrum and tailbone backward to increase space front to back

EXERCISES TO OPEN THE PELVIC OUTLET

Preparing to open the pelvic outlet is a similar approach to the lower midpelvis, where you try to achieve internal rotation and adduction at the hip and a posterior pelvic tilt. Plus, it's beneficial to strengthen the lats to influence the sacral position and generate power while pushing. Exercises that emphasize outlet opening include hip hinge exercises, such as deadlifts and staggered stance RDLs, and horizontal rows, such as bent-over rows or single-arm rows.

PELVIC OUTLET OPENING EXERCISES: INTERNAL ROTATION WITH ADDUCTION AND POSTERIOR TILT (KNEES IN, ANKLES OUT)

STRENGTHENING EXERCISES	MOBILITY EXERCISES
Deadlifts	Forward-leaning lat release
Closed hip at the bottom of:	Standing lat release
• Lunges	Half-kneeling hip flexor release
• Split squats	Couch stretch
• Step-ups	Hip-shifted breathing drills
Staggered-stance RDL	Pelvic floor releases
Single-leg deadlift	Back expansion breathing drills
Poor man's leg curl	
Good mornings	

PELVIC OUTLET OPENING EXERCISES: LAT ENGAGEMENT FOR NEUTRAL SPINE AND SACRAL TRACTION

STRENGTHENING EXERCISES	MOBILITY EXERCISES
Bent-over rows	Pelvic mobility: Cat/cows
Single-arm row	Chest mobility: Floor or wall angels
Lat pull-downs	Thoracic mobility: Side-seated side-body opener
Ring rows	Sacral tuberous release
Inverted rows	

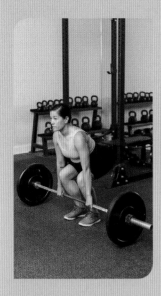
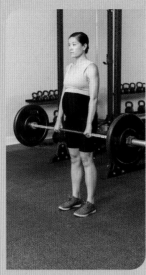

HIP HINGE EXERCISES AND DEADLIFTS

The hamstrings play a prominent role in pulling the pelvis into internal rotation and a posterior tilt, to create space in the lower half of the pelvis. Hip hinge–focused exercises have more hip flexion than knee flexion and will affect the hamstrings more than the quadriceps.

The deadlift is a compound exercise that works several muscle groups in the upper and lower body, including the hamstrings, adductors, and latissimus dorsi. It's essential to strengthen these muscles when opening the pelvic outlet and pushing during labor.

POOR MAN'S LEG CURL

The poor man's leg curl is a body weight hamstring strengthening exercise. You can do this movement with one or both legs. The key is to drive the heel into the elevated surface to activate the hamstrings.

1 Starting in a supine position, place one or both heels onto an elevated surface, such as a couch or bench.

2 Exhale to drive through the heel(s) to lift the hips toward the ceiling. As you drive the hips up, focus on pushing the hips toward the ceiling, and tuck the butt under at the top of the movement.

3 Maintain this position for 2 to 5 seconds.

4 Inhale to slowly lower to the bottom of the movement.

5 Repeat 10 to 20 times. If doing one leg, repeat on the other leg.

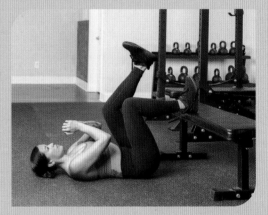
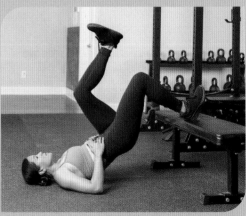

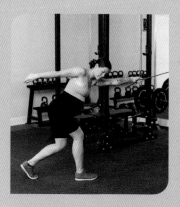 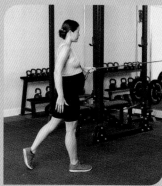

STAGGERED-STANCE DEADLIFT WITH BANDED ROW

The staggered-stance deadlift can be done with a weight or band. This exercise is a posterior oblique sling–focused exercise that strengthens the hamstring, adductor, and glute with the hip hinge. You can review the weighted variation of this movement on page 121.

The banded variation of the staggered stance deadlift allows you to maintain a more upright position that could accommodate for your growing belly, while still emphasizing internal rotation at the hip.

1 Start in a staggered-stance position, with one leg forward and the other foot slightly behind you. Hold the band in the hand opposite of the forward leg.

2 Inhale to lower to the bottom of the deadlift as you reach forward with the band.

3 As you lower, rotate the belly toward your thigh to find internal rotation at the hip. You should feel more of a stretching sensation in the glute and hamstring of the forward leg.

4 Keep weight in the big toe of the forward leg and keep the forward knee aligned over the ankle.

5 Exhale to stand up as you extend in the hip and row the band back as you stand up.

6 At the top, find an open hip position.

7 Repeat 10 times per side.

BENT-OVER ROWS

The lats influence the sacral position and help you generate power while pushing. Bent-over rows and other horizontal pulling exercises strengthen the lats from a lengthened to a shortened position. Bent-over rows can be done with a barbell or dumbbell, using either one or both arms.

If you need more support at the bottom of the movement, lower the weights to an elevated surface, such as a box, or adjust to a seated position with bands or cable machines.

SAMPLE PELVIC OUTLET-OPENING WORKOUT

Here is a sample workout that you could incorporate once a week as a part of your birth preparation. This exercise incorporates movement patterns required to open the bottom part of the pelvis.

MOBILITY	3 ROUNDS
• 30 seconds per side of supported standing hip shift • 30 seconds per side of forward-leaning lat release • 30 seconds per side of half-kneeling hip flexor release	• 10 repetitions of deadlift • 10 repetitions per side of staggered-stance deadlift with banded row • 10 repetitions per side of single-arm row

PREPARING YOUR BABY FOR BIRTH

Now that you understand the different exercises you can incorporate into your workout routine to prepare to open the pelvis for birth, let's explore how movement can prepare your baby for birth as well. There is no one perfect position for your baby during labor. Each pelvic level is shaped differently, so your baby must rotate through several positions to fit into each part of the pelvis.

Depending on how far you've ventured into birth research and explored birth forums, you may have encountered the notion that there's a single optimal position for your baby for birth. Your provider may have even mentioned that "your baby is in the best position for birth," often referring to when the back of the head is positioned directly at the front of the pelvis or oriented toward the front-left side of the pelvis. However, your baby needs to rotate through several positions, so there isn't a single "best" position. The "best" position is one in which your baby tucks their chin to their chest and presents the smallest, and this may be on either side.

THE MAMASTEFIT BIRTH PREPARATION CIRCUIT

The MamasteFit birth preparation circuit focuses on releasing common areas of prenatal tension, which can make it easier for your baby to rotate and move through the pelvis. This circuit makes an internal rotation with adduction at the hip and a posterior pelvic tilt easier to achieve while releasing tension in the posterior pelvic floor. I recommend incorporating this series into your weekly routine 2 to 4 times a week after 20 weeks of pregnancy.

The circuit includes:

- **Forward-leaning inversion:** Releases lower uterine ligaments to support baby's head position

- **Back expansion breathing drill:** Positioning the thoracic spine in flexion enables us to leverage our breathing mechanics to alleviate any limitations or tightness in the back

- **Forward-leaning lat release:** Stretches the shortened latissimus dorsi muscle to support finding a posterior pelvic tilt and rounding in the posterior chain

- **Half-kneeling hip flexor release with side opener:** Stretches the hip flexor muscles to support finding a posterior pelvic tilt and releasing in the side of the body

- **Hip-shifted pelvic tilts:** Spinal and pelvic mobility with asymmetrical positioning to release the contralateral anterior and posterior pelvic floor; this movement also orients one-half of the pelvis into internal rotation

- **Supported standing hip shift:** Positions the pelvis into an asymmetrical opening of the contralateral anterior and posterior pelvic quadrants and releases the posterior pelvic floor; this movement also orients one-half of the pelvis into internal rotation

FORWARD-LEANING INVERSION

The first movement focuses on releasing uterine ligament tension. The uterine ligaments can influence the uterine shape, which could support or hinder your baby's position. The forward-leaning inversion positions your head below your hips, using gravity to stretch and untwist the lower uterine ligaments and vertically oriented round ligaments.

1 Start in an upright position with hip extended on an elevated surface, such as your couch.

2 Carefully move to place your forearms on the floor in an inverted position. The inversion should be fairly upright; legs should be relaxed. Your partner can spot you in this position by placing their hands under your shoulders.

3 Tuck the chin to chest.

4 Hold this position for 3 full cycles of breath.

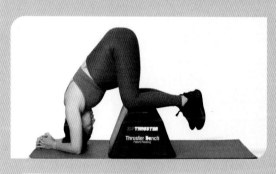

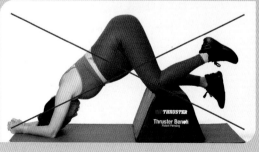

You may feel a stretching sensation in the lower back and sacral area and in the lower abdomen. If you feel lightheaded or dizzy, bring your knees to the floor and rest before standing up. If you have elevated blood pressure or hypertension, you may want to avoid inversions.

What if this movement is too intense for you? Try a less-intense inversion variation, such as puppy pose or open-knee chest.

The next three movements of the circuit focus on increasing the range of motion of the rib cage, spine, and pelvis to achieve more of a posterior pelvic tilt, which opens the pelvic inlet.

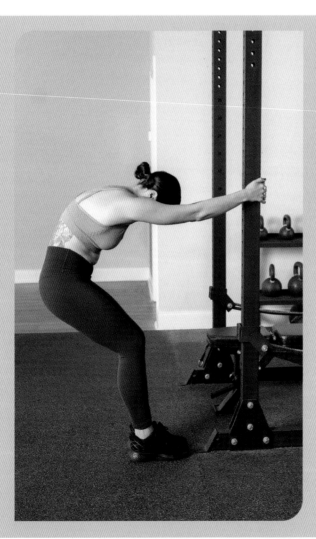

BACK EXPANSION BREATHING DRILL

In this exercise, you round your back, which counteracts the typical prenatal posture. This breathing technique is designed to reconfigure your breathing mechanics, facilitating the expansion of the thoracic cavity.

1 Start in a standing position and grab onto a sturdy structure about an arm's length away, such as a door frame.

2 Sink back into your heels and hips as you round in the back.

3 Inhale to feel an increased pressure in your back.

4 Exhale to pull the rib cage and pelvis closer together on the front side of the body to deepen the rounded position.

5 Breathe here for 5 to 10 full breath cycles.

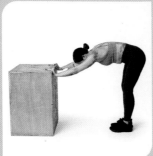

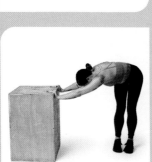

FORWARD-LEANING LAT RELEASE

This exercise supports rib cage and pelvic positioning by addressing tightness or restriction in the lats, which facilitates the opening of the pelvic levels during labor.

1 Start by pressing your hands into a wall as you hinge the hips back.

2 Then step the feet perpendicular to the hands, forming a 90-degree angle.

3 This will increase the stretching sensation of the side of your body on the lengthened side.

4 Press harder into the stretched side's hand to intensify the stretch.

5 Push the chest and belly away from the floor to find a slight rounding in the back; this will intensify the release sensation.

6 Hold for 5 to 10 full breath cycles, then switch sides.

HALF-KNEELING HIP FLEXOR RELEASE WITH SIDE OPENER

This exercise releases the hip flexor muscles that pull the pelvis into an anterior pelvic tilt, which increases the range of motion of the pelvic position and makes it easier to find a posterior pelvic tilt.

1 Start in a half-kneeling position.

2 Tuck the butt underneath to feel a stretch in the front side of the pelvis.

3 Maintain this tucked position as you gradually push the hips forward.

4 Reach up and overhead with the same-side arm, creating a stretch in the side of the body and lats.

5 Rotate the chest toward the floor, forward, and toward the ceiling to adjust the sensation in the side of the body.

6 Hold this position for 5 to 10 full breath cycles, then switch to the other side.

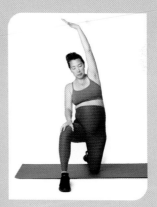

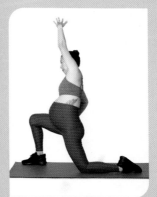

HIP-SHIFTED PELVIC TILTS

In the final two movements of the MamasteFit birth prep circuit, the primary emphasis is on internally rotating the hip and releasing tension in the posterior pelvic floor.

The hip-shifted pelvic tilt is a unilateral pelvic tilting movement. This movement adjusts the pelvic position and releases tension in the posterior pelvic floor, supporting the opening of the midpelvis. In this pelvic tilting variation, the elevated hip is forced into internal rotation as the lower hip is in external rotation, which creates more of a release than if you had the hips even with one another.

1 Start in a tabletop position.

2 Elevate one knee on a yoga block or 2- to 3-inch (5–8-cm)–high surface

3 Shift weight toward the elevated knee, adjusting your hand position as needed. If this is difficult, push the down knee into a wall to push your weight toward the elevated knee. When doing this, ensure the down knee is lower than the elevated knee.

4 Push the chest and belly away from the floor to round in the back, feeling more of a sensation in the lower back of the elevated hip.

5 Hold here for a full breath cycle.

6 Then drop the belly to the floor to arch in the back, feeling more of a sensation in the lower abdomen of the lower hip.

7 Repeat for a total of 5 to 10 pelvic tilts, then switch sides.

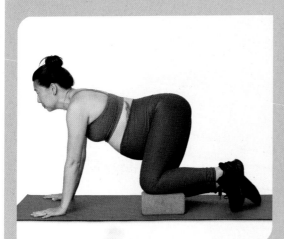

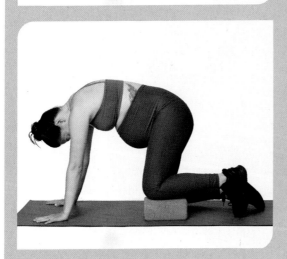

SUPPORTED STANDING HIP SHIFT

This exercise positions the pelvis in an asymmetrical opening to prompt internal rotation and release tension in the posterior pelvic floor, similar to the previous standing hip shifts. In this variation, you are also incorporating a lat release.

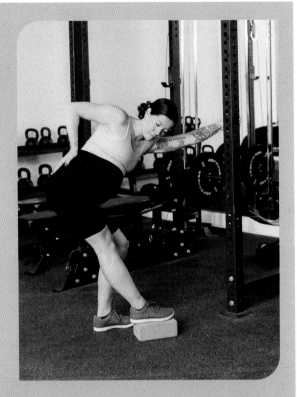

1 Standing roughly arm's length from a sturdy structure. You may need to move a little closer or further after you've shifted into the position.

2 Place one foot elevated on a yoga block or 2- to 3-inch (5–8-cm)–high surface.

3 Grab onto a sturdy structure with the hand opposite to the elevated hip.

4 Hinge the hips back to straighten the supporting arm. You should feel a stretch in the supporting arm.

5 Shift weight toward the elevated foot as you straighten the leg.

6 Rotate the belly toward your thigh, keeping your weight on the big toe.

7 Push the belly and chest away from the floor as you round in the back to increase the sensation in the back and posterior pelvic floor of the elevated side.

8 Breathe here for 5 to 10 full cycles of breath, then switch sides

LABOR PREPARATION

You can prepare for birth by practicing labor positions and comfort measures either with your partner or solo. Practicing during pregnancy will help you identify which positions feel comfortable and restorative for you. In the last few weeks of pregnancy, you can incorporate labor preparation workouts 1 or 2 times a week to rehearse for your birth.

LABOR PREPARATION WORKOUT

5 to 10 rounds of:

- 15 to 20 seconds of aerobic exercise to increase heart rate and respiration rate, and to generate exercise-induced stress, followed immediately by:
- 1 to 2 minutes of relaxing into a labor position and implementing a comfort measure (choose positions from the list below and see examples in chapter 8)

INLET OPENING-FOCUSED WORKOUT

These labor positions tend to open the top of the pelvis and are focused on front-to-back movement patterns that emphasize external rotation of the femurs and pelvic tilting. Explore which positions feel the easiest for you to relax and which are most accessible for you.

- Standing rocks/pelvic tilts
- Leaning rocks/pelvic tilts
- Supported squats (partner, long fabric, or sturdy structure)
- Seated pelvic tilts (birth ball)
- All-fours rocks (birth ball)

MIDPELVIS OPENING-FOCUSED WORKOUT

These labor positions tend to open the midpelvis with side-to-side and asymmetrical movement patterns. Explore which positions feel easier to relax and which are most accessible for you.

- Standing sway
- Elevated-side lunge
- Leaning sway
- Seated hip circles
- Seated hip sways
- All-fours hip sways (Option to elevate one knee with a yoga block)
- Half-kneeling lunge

COUNTERPRESSURE-FOCUSED WORKOUT

Choose a variety of positions and explore which counterpressure techniques feel the best and are accessible in each position.

- Double hip squeeze
- Pelvic press
- Sacral counter pressure

BIRTH BALL-FOCUSED WORKOUT

All positions are supported by a birth or stability ball. Most birth locations will have a birth ball available in their labor suites.

- Seated pelvic tilts
- Seated hip circles
- All-fours rocks
- All-fours hip sways
- Half-lunge rocks

Labor preparation workouts create exercise-induced stress to replicate the physiological response of contractions during labor. This is followed by a dedicated period of 1 to 2 minutes where you prioritize activating your parasympathetic nervous system by relaxing in a labor position with a labor comfort technique. Chapter 8 discusses labor positions and comfort techniques in more detail.

PREPARING FOR A SCHEDULED CESAREAN

A 2021 CDC report listed the U.S. Cesarean birth rate at 32.1 percent. Some Cesareans are scheduled, while many others result from labor complications. If you are scheduling a Cesarean birth, preparing for that procedure can be incorporated into prenatal workouts.

Preparing for a Cesarean birth includes:

- Spinal flexion
- Anterior oblique sling neuromuscular connection

Spinal Flexion: Preparation for Epidural or Spinal

Anesthesia is a key component of a Cesarean birth. The anesthesiologist or certified registered nurse anesthetist (CRNA) administers regional anesthesia, such as a spinal, epidural, or combination of the two, into the back to block pain during birth. Spinal flexion, or rounding the spine forward, opens up space between the vertebrae to allow greater ease of catheter (spinal or epidural) placement.

Some exercises you can include in your preparation are:

- Lat and hip flexor mobility (included in the birth prep circuit)
- Pelvic tilts, both unilaterally and bilaterally (pages 34)
- Back expansion breathing drills (included in the birth prep circuit)

You can incorporate the lat release, hip flexor release, and back expansion exercises from prior portions of this chapter, including the MamasteFit birth preparation circuit. Symmetrical pelvic tilts can be performed seated, which most closely replicates spinal or epidural placement. Asymmetrical pelvic tilts isolate one side of the pelvis at a time, facilitating opening in whichever side is more restricted.

Anterior Oblique Sling

Next, you can focus on integrating the anterior oblique sling as a part of your Cesarean birth preparation. The benefit of prenatal exercise extends beyond birth to postpartum recovery. Developing a neuromuscular connection with exercises preoperatively is an effective and commonly used rehabilitation strategy.

The anterior oblique sling is a myofascial sling that runs from the chest to the opposite adductor, as we discussed in chapter 5 (page 87). This sling crosses the lower abdomen where a C-section incision is made. This sling is cut during the Cesarean birth, contributing to a severed disconnection with your core. Creating familiar demand for the anterior oblique sling can hasten your return to function and fitness as the tissues heal and become safe to activate. See chapter 9 for more guidance on C-section recovery after birth.

KEY TAKEAWAYS

Your prenatal workouts can do more than just keep you strong and comfortable throughout your pregnancy—they can also prepare you for birth. You can incorporate pelvic opening exercises to ensure that you can easily open each pelvic level, as a big reason for labor stalls is the decreased movement capability of the pelvis. Alleviating common areas of tension during pregnancy can make it easier for your baby to navigate the pelvis during labor.

PART 3

BIRTH

THE FINAL PART OF PREGNANCY IS BIRTH—this is the final step before you meet your baby!

This section provides tangible tools, such as labor positions and comfort measures, for you and your birth partner to utilize during your labor, with an understanding of *when* to use these tools. Plus, you'll learn how to resolve issues during your labor with movement techniques, many of which you've learned in part 2 of the book. While this book does not provide in-depth childbirth education, the tools you'll gather from this section will increase your confidence and improve your birth experience.

EIGHT
LABOR

IN THIS CHAPTER, WE WILL BE COVERING labor positions and comfort measures that you can practice in advance and utilize during your labor to have a more positive birth experience. You've already learned many of the physiological terms and useful exercises these techniques are based on in earlier sections of this book, so if you've been working out and following the routines I describe here, you'll be in great shape and able to tolerate the demands of birth.

Birth is impossible to predict, but that doesn't mean you shouldn't plan for it or share your preferences with your birth team. Rather, understand that you may have to adjust your plan while in labor. Think of this mindset as an extension of the adaptability and flexibility practiced throughout pregnancy with your prenatal workouts.

Let's start by discussing what the best labor position is for your birth, and how each position can influence the space in your pelvis.

LABOR POSITIONS

The best labor position is the one that creates more space in the specific part of the pelvis that your baby is currently trying to navigate. You can figure out where your baby is in your pelvis by understanding fetal station, or where the baby is in your pelvis.

FETAL STATION

Fetal station is how high or low the baby is within your pelvis. It is measured by where your baby is compared to a bony bump in the pelvis called the ischial spine. If your baby is above the ischial spine, it's a minus station (like –1). If your baby is at the ischial spine, that's a 0 station. When your baby is below, it's a plus station (like +1). These stations roughly correlate to the pelvic inlet, midpelvis, and pelvic outlet, each of which opens with different types of movement patterns and labor positions (see chapter 7, page 110).

A labor position should optimize space in the specific part of your pelvis that your baby is presently passing through, making it easier for them to engage, rotate, and exit the pelvis comfortably, which may or may not correlate to a specific phase of labor.

You can learn your baby's station by:

- Paying attention to your body's natural movements during contractions. You tend to intuitively make more space in your pelvis for your baby as you work through contractions.

- Your provider or nurse can use a cervical exam to determine your baby's station.

Intuitive Movement Patterns

During labor, you tend to intuitively move to create the necessary space for your baby. This innate connection to the birthing process is often more noticeable when you're unmedicated. However, it's possible to maintain this connection even if you have an epidural.

When your baby is positioned higher in the pelvis, you naturally favor labor positions that open up the top of your pelvis. As your baby enters the pelvis, you'll favor movements that open the middle of the pelvis. And this pattern continues when your baby is low in the pelvis.

MOVEMENT PATTERNS BY BABY POSITION

BABY POSITION IN PELVIS	MOVEMENT PATTERNS TO FAVOR
High in pelvis	Front-to-back movements Pelvic tilting or rocking "Tucky" movements (repeatedly tucking butt under)
Engaged in midpelvis	Side-to-side movements Hip-shifted movements Asymmetrical or diagonal movements
Low in pelvis (pushing)	Mini or quarter squats Knees in closer to ankles Coming up on your tippy toes

If you and your partner pay attention to your movement patterns during contractions, it can be a clue to where your baby is in the pelvis.

A simple way to remember is:

- **If your baby is high,** you tend to favor front-to-back type movements.

- **If your baby has already engaged,** you'll likely favor side-to-side or swaying motions.

- **When your baby is low in the pelvis,** you might naturally feel the urge to start pushing, which makes it quite clear where your baby is in your pelvis.

Recognizing these movement patterns can guide you to choose labor positions that best support your birth.

PELVIC INLET: HELPING YOUR BABY ENGAGE

Starting at the top of the pelvis, your baby attempts to enter and engage in the pelvic inlet. Your baby is in the process of rotating to match the shape of the upper pelvis while tucking their chin to their chest to present a smaller profile to the pelvis. Wider knees, deep squats, and front-to-back pelvic tilting help open up the top part of the pelvis, making it easier for your baby to enter and engage into the pelvic inlet.

MOVEMENT PATTERNS THAT OPEN THE PELVIC INLET

BIOMECHANICAL PATTERN	WHAT IT LOOKS LIKE	WHAT IT DOES
External rotation of the femurs with abduction	Knees out, ankles in	Creates more space side to side
Posterior pelvic tilt	Tucking the butt underneath	Creates more space front to back
Anterior pelvic tilt	Arching in the back	Makes external rotation easier, which can create more space side to side Changes pubic bone angle

Pelvic inlet opening labor positions include:

- Supported squats
- Seated pelvic tilts on a birth ball
- All-fours pelvic tilts with a birth ball
- Wide knees with a peanut ball (this is a birth ball that is peanut-shaped)

During contractions, choose one of these positions to create space in the top of your pelvis. Between contractions, choose a comfortable position to rest, like sitting or lying, or stay in the labor position. Maintain the same position for as long as it's comfortable (often 30 to 45 minutes before switching).

SEATED PELVIC TILTS

Seated pelvic tilts can be done on a chair or couch, but are easiest on a birth ball. Most birth locations have birth balls available, but they are worth investing in for home use.

Your partner can position themselves to provide physical support as you rock your hips forward and backward. Have them stand behind you, or sit in front where you can lean on them.

1 During contractions, rock hips forward and backward.

2 As you rock your hips forward, round your back.

3 As you rock your hips backward, arch your back.

4 You can widen the knees as you rock your hips forward and backward.

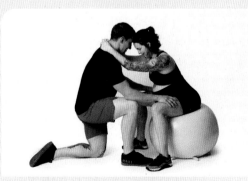

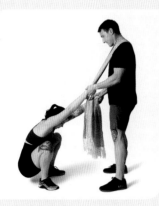 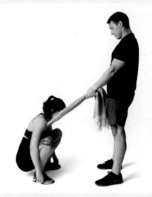 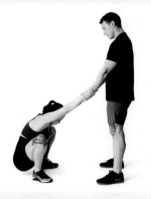

SUPPORTED SQUATS

Supported squats help open the top of the pelvis. It is essential to relax your legs and release into the position. This is why a supported position is essential! There are a number of support options, like hanging a long sheet over a doorframe, routing a long sheet behind your partner's back, routing a long sheet under your arms, or holding onto your partners' hands. Keep your feet flat on the floor, knees wide, legs relaxed, and back rounded.

1 Choose support variation.

2 Lower to the bottom of the squat.

3 Move as comfortable in this position.

4 **Two options:** Maintain squat throughout the contraction, then your partner can assist you to stand between contractions. Alternatively, maintain the squat during and between contractions.

ALL-FOURS PELVIC TILTS

The wide-knee position in the all-fours pelvic tilt will create space side to side in the top of the pelvis. In this position, your birth partner can apply counterpressure behind you or sit in front of you to speak words of affirmation, hold your hands, or massage your shoulders and scalp.

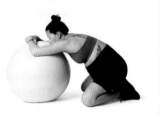

1 Begin in a tabletop position, with your chest leaning on a supportive surface like a birth ball.

2 Rock your hips forward and backward.

3 As you rock forward, arch your back.

4 As you rock backward, round your back.

5 Move through a range of motion that feels comfortable for you.

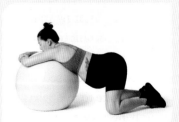

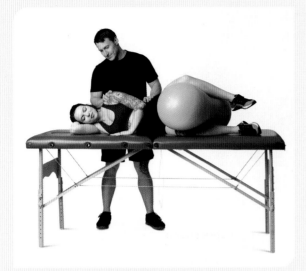
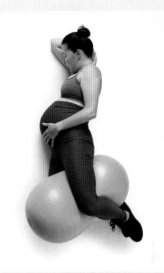

WIDE KNEES WITH PEANUT BALL

If you want to rest or have restricted mobility from an epidural, using a peanut ball can be helpful to open the pelvis. You can also use two or three pillows in the same way to create space.

1 Place the peanut ball between the knees to spread the knees apart to create external rotation at the hip.

2 Keep the knees forward, with the ball between the knees.

3 Rest on your side for 20 to 30 minutes, then switch sides.

Another option is to fully extend your hip without arching the back. In this position, the full hip extension tucks the pelvis underneath, creating a posterior pelvic tilt. You can rest in this hip-extended position for 20 to 30 minutes, then switch sides.

MIDPELVIS: HELPING YOUR BABY ROTATE

The next level of the pelvis that your baby is going to move through is the midpelvis. You may intuitively favor side-to-side or swaying-type movements during your contractions, indicating your baby has engaged in the pelvis and is beginning to rotate.

It's important to address the common misconception that the best labor position corresponds directly with your phase of labor. Early labor doesn't always mean you should be focused on pelvic inlet opening, and active labor doesn't necessarily equate to midpelvis opening movements. Choose labor positions based on your baby's position instead. You might find yourself in early labor but primarily engaging in midpelvis opening movements because your baby is already engaged, or conversely, you could be in active labor while still emphasizing inlet opening movements because your baby hasn't fully engaged in the pelvis.

The midpelvis itself can be further divided into two sections: the upper and lower parts. The upper midpelvis opens up like the pelvic inlet, but it's just on one side. On the other hand, the lower midpelvis opens up more like the pelvic outlet, but again, it's one-sided. This means that the entire midpelvis tends to open up more effectively with side-to-side or swaying types of movements. Let's break down each section of the midpelvis.

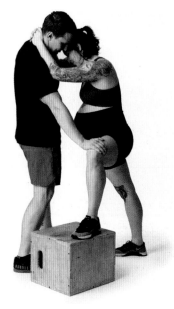

Upper Midpelvis

The top half of the midpelvis is the upper midpelvis; this is where your baby begins their rotation after engaging into the pelvic inlet. You may favor more open hip positions, where your knee is away from the center of your body, such as an elevated lunge.

To create more space in the upper midpelvis, use movement patterns that resemble those of the pelvic inlet but that primarily happen on one side. So, you might find yourself leaning toward a one-sided elevated lunge instead of adopting a deep squat position.

Lower Midpelvis

The bottom half of the midpelvis is the lower midpelvis; this is where your baby finishes their rotation to get under the pubic bone. You may favor shifting your weight repeatedly into the same leg, as weight bearing tends to open the lower midpelvis more with internal rotation and adduction at the hip, meaning the leg rotates inward and moves closer to the center of your body.

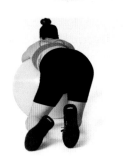

The lower midpelvis is more receptive to closed hip positions, or movement patterns that imitate the pelvic outlet. Just like the upper midpelvis, these movements predominantly occur on one side. Consequently, you might naturally lean toward a posterior pelvic tilt on one side because the position of your pelvis significantly influences your ability to achieve internal or external hip rotation.

If you're finding it challenging to picture this, take a look at the all-fours hip shift with a yoga block. In this particular labor position, the hip that's raised on the yoga block is in a closed hip position, which opens the lower midpelvis.

Midpelvis opening labor positions include:

- Standing sway
- Elevated lunge
- Curb walking or sideways stairs
- Seated sway or hip circles
- Half-lunge with birth ball
- All-fours sway with birth ball
- Side-lying with partner supported rock

MOVEMENT PATTERNS THAT OPEN THE UPPER MIDPELVIS (ONE-SIDED)

BIOMECHANICAL PATTERN	WHAT IT LOOKS LIKE	WHAT IT DOES
External rotation of the femurs with abduction	Open hip positions One leg in a wide-legged position	Creates more space one-sided in the upper half of the pelvis to make it easier for your baby to begin their rotation
Anterior pelvic tilt	Arching in the back	Makes external rotation easier, which can increase the space available

MOVEMENT PATTERNS THAT OPEN THE LOWER MIDPELVIS (ONE-SIDED)

BIOMECHANICAL PATTERN	WHAT IT LOOKS LIKE	WHAT IT DOES
External rotation of the femurs with abduction	Knee in, ankle out Closed hip positions Putting weight into one leg	Creates more space one-sided in the lower half of your pelvis to make it easier for your baby to finish their rotation under the pubic bone
Posterior pelvic tilt	Tucking the butt under Rounded back	Makes it easier to find internal rotation, which can increase the space available

During contractions, you can choose from any of those labor positions to help create space within the middle of your pelvis. Between contractions, you can opt for a comfortable resting position, such as sitting, on all fours, or lying down, or you can maintain the labor position you were in during contractions. You can stick with the same labor position as long as it remains comfortable for you, which might typically be 30 to 45 minutes before you feel the need to switch to a different position.

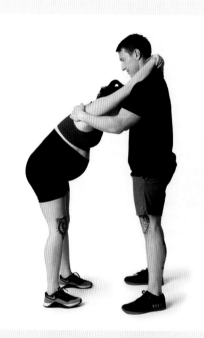

ELEVATED LUNGE

In this position, you place one foot on an elevated surface as you open the hip, which helps open the upper midpelvis, as the leg opens away from the midline. Your partner can stand in front of you as you lean into them, and they can press your knee out further as you rock into the leg to increase space in the upper midpelvis.

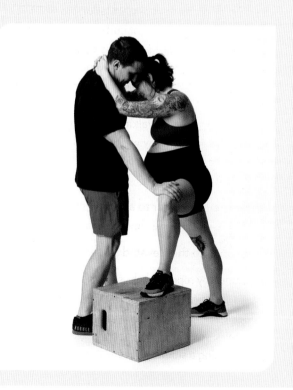

STANDING SWAY

This position involves leaning on your partner, a countertop or elevated surface, or standing without support as you sway your hips from side to side. You can also shift your weight from leg to leg or emphasize a hip shift as you sway. The repetitive sway alternates the opening of the upper and lower midpelvis, helping your baby rock and rotate through the midpelvis.

UPRIGHT LABOR POSITIONS

Upright labor positions and movement increase pressure on the cervix due to gravity. This increased pressure can speed up the labor feedback loop and decrease the length of your labor! This is the main reason why exercising during pregnancy can decrease the length of your labor—you have the stamina and strength to maintain an upright position and move longer if you are in good physical condition.

CURB WALKING OR SIDEWAYS STAIRS

Curb walking is a technique where you walk with one foot on an elevated surface, like a sidewalk curb, and the other foot on a lower surface, such as the road. Curb walking is often recommended as a way to encourage your baby to engage and possibly initiate labor. You might come across it in lists of exercises that are suggested to kick-start labor. However, it's essential to understand that curb walking primarily focuses on opening the midpelvis by emphasizing hip hiking and an asymmetrical stance. Unfortunately, there isn't a guaranteed movement that can reliably trigger the onset of labor.

In addition to curb walking, you can achieve a similar pelvic opening by walking up stairs sideways. Here are some tips for both curb walking and sideways stairs:

1 Stand perpendicular to an elevated ledge or stair, with one foot on the elevated surface.

2 Step up onto the elevated surface.

3 Continue by repeating these steps for additional steps or stairs. If you're curb walking, you'll keep moving forward along the curb. If you're walking up stairs, you'll continue to ascend the stairs while maintaining a sideways orientation.

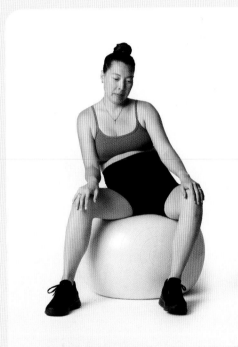

SEATED SWAY OR HIP CIRCLES

If you need more support in your labor position, you can sit on a birth ball and gently sway your hips from side to side or move them in a circular motion.

HALF LUNGE WITH BIRTH BALL

In a half lunge position, place your chest or forearms on a birth ball for support and place one leg forward, the other with knee down behind you. During contractions, gently rock diagonally into the forward leg for added comfort and relief. Place a pad or pillow under the knee on the ground to enhance your comfort during this position.

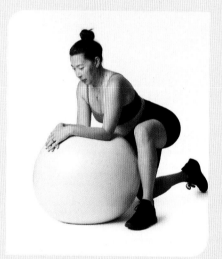

ALL-FOURS SWAY WITH BIRTH BALL

This position resembles the pelvic inlet opening variations, but here your hips move from side to side rather than front to back. Place your chest against the birth ball and gently sway your hips in a side-to-side motion, which creates an asymmetrical space in the midpelvis.

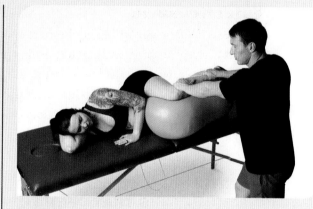

SIDE-LYING WITH PARTNER-SUPPORTED ROCK

This is a great option for incorporating movement and opening the midpelvis if you need to rest or have an epidural.

1 Lying on your side, rest the bottom leg slightly behind you.

2 Place a peanut ball under the top leg, supporting the knee and ankle on the ball.

3 When a contraction begins, your partner will gently pull the top leg forward to open the hip, creating space in the upper midpelvis.

4 Subsequently, your partner will push the leg backward to close the hip, making room in the lower midpelvis.

5 Continue this rocking motion back and forth throughout the entire duration of the contraction.

6 Between contractions, your partner can provide massages or gentle jiggling to help you relax further.

Repeat this process during contractions for 30 to 45 minutes, then switch sides. This position and rocking movement facilitate an asymmetrical space in your midpelvis, aiding your baby in rocking and rotating through this area.

PELVIC OUTLET: PUSHING

As you near the end of labor, you will either begin to spontaneously push or receive guidance to start actively pushing. During the pushing phase, the emphasis is on opening the pelvic outlet, which is the lower part of the pelvis. This involves three main movements: internal rotation and adduction at the hip, keeping a neutral spine with a slight tilt, and sacral nutation. Let's explore how to use these movements in your pushing positions.

MOVEMENT PATTERNS THAT OPEN THE PELVIC OUTLET

BIOMECHANICAL PATTERN	WHAT IT LOOKS LIKE	WHAT IT DOES
Internal rotation and adduction at the femur	Knees in, ankles out	Spreads the sitz bones further apart to create more space side to side in the pelvic outlet
Neutral spine with a slight posterior pelvic tilt	Flat back, rib cage stacked over the pelvis	Increases the strength of your pushes and the slight posterior pelvic tilt makes internal rotation easier, so it can increase space side to side
Sacral nutation	The movement of the sacrum may not be observable from the outside Lat engagement can encourage the sacrum to shift in this direction, along with the maintaining a position that allows the sacrum to move freely by avoiding lying flat on your back	The sacrum tilts forward and downward, moving the bottom of the sacrum backward This creates more space from front to back in the pelvic outlet

The bottom of the pelvis opens more with internal rotation and adduction at the hip, or knees in and ankles out. This knees-in-and-ankles-out position can be done in really any position: supine, side-lying, all fours, and even standing.

Pelvic outlet opening labor positions include:

- Side-lying with partner support
- All fours with knees in
- Outlet-opening peanut ball resting position
- Supine with pillow support
- Sacral tuberous release

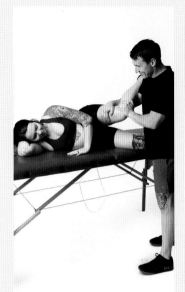

SIDE-LYING WITH PARTNER SUPPORT

The side-lying position is a great pushing position for both unmedicated and epidural births. This position is restful, so it helps you relax more between pushes. Additionally, your sacrum has plenty of space and your partner can support your leg in internal rotation to increase space in the pelvic outlet.

1 Start on either side, although you may find that you prefer one side over the other.

2 Your partner routes their arm under your lower leg, resting your lower leg on their forearm, and places their hand on your thigh.

3 When your partner lifts their forearm, your leg will internally rotate.

4 During pushes, your partner will gently rotate your leg as you push.

OUTLET-OPENING PEANUT BALL RESTING POSITION

In between pushing, you can place a ball between your ankles to open the bottom of the pelvis as you rest. This prompts internal rotation at the hip, which creates more space side to side in the bottom of the pelvis. This position may not be appropriate to actually push in, but it can be a great resting position.

Pushing during labor is essentially a pressure management activity, and the goal is to increase pressure within the abdominal cavity to assist with pushing your baby out. Pushing is a coordinated effort that involves more than simply contracting your abdominal muscles to push the baby out. It's important to understand that your pelvic floor doesn't push the baby out; it simply needs to move out of the way for your baby while pushing.

A helpful analogy is to think of squeezing a tube of toothpaste: If you squeeze from the sides (engaging your abdominal muscles), the toothpaste will come out, but it might not be as efficient or effective as pushing from the top of the tube (using your diaphragm). In this way, focusing on pressure management and optimal alignment can enhance your pushing efforts during labor.

Another consideration for creating more space in the pelvic outlet is the position of the sacrum. You want to use a position that allows the sacrum to move as your baby pushes through. This may include not pushing flat on your back and adding some pillows under your hips to create space.

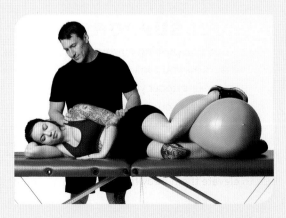

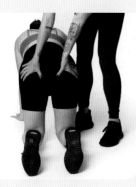 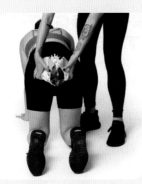 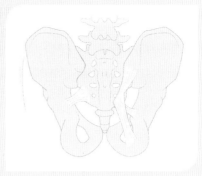

SACRAL TUBEROUS RELEASE

If your sacrum feels "stuck," your partner can do a sacral tuberous release to ease tension in the ligaments that attach to your sacrum. This can be done between pushes, or while you are laboring down and waiting to push.

1 In a side-lying or all-fours position, identify the landmarks of the tailbone and the sitz bone. These three points should form a triangle.

2 In the middle of the two sides of the triangle, you'll find the sacral tuberous ligament. Your partner should place their thumbs in these spaces.

3 You can cough or laugh, and your partner will feel these ligaments tighten under

their thumbs, confirming they are in the correct locations.

4 Your partner can gently massage this area to release tension. This should provide a sensation of relief and relaxation.

Additionally, lat engagement, or pulling on your legs, bed handles, or a sheet can facilitate sacral nutation. This movement tilts the bottom of your sacrum backward, creating additional space in the pelvic outlet. As you pull, keep your elbows in and your palms up, which tends to engage the lats more to influence the sacral position. Avoid having your elbows flare out or using an overhand grip, as this may shift the engagement toward the shoulders and upper back.

SUPINE WITH PILLOW SUPPORT

If you do find that pushing on your back feels best for you, you can place pillows or rolled-up blankets under your hips or back to create space for your sacrum. You might place a pillow along one side of your back to tilt you to the side slightly, or you can place two pillows or blankets under your hips to elevate them away from the bed.

ALL FOURS WITH KNEES IN

The all-fours position is an upright option that uses gravity to aid in pushing. Upright positions are more active and can be tiring. You can use the all-fours position whether you have an unmedicated birth or an epidural, provided you have the mobility and support from your health care provider. In a tabletop position, slightly widen your ankles compared to your knees to help create more space in the pelvic outlet as you push.

There is no single best labor position because no single position can open the entire pelvis. The key is to concentrate on creating space in the specific part of the pelvis your baby is currently navigating. If your baby is still high and attempting to engage, you can create more space in the upper pelvis by widening your knees and using pelvic tilting movements. When your baby is engaged and rotating through the pelvis, creating space in the midpelvis with side-to-side and swaying motions can be helpful. During the pushing stage, look for positions that maximize space in the pelvic outlet.

Now, let's explore some techniques to help yourself feel more comfortable during labor.

COMFORT MEASURES: COUNTERPESSURE

Comfort measures can—and should—be incorporated during early labor, active labor, or even while pushing. In fact, during early labor, it's a good idea to practice some comfort measures to determine which ones you prefer while your contractions are still manageable. This way, it becomes easier to choose the ones that provide the most relief during the more intense stages of labor. You can even practice these techniques during your pregnancy.

Comfort measures encompass a range of methods you or your partner can use to reduce the intensity and discomfort of your contractions. By introducing pleasurable stimuli, such as counterpressure, it's possible to diminish the sensation of pain. The primary aim of comfort measures is to help you relax more during contractions, which can contribute to a quicker labor progression. Hydrotherapy, aromatherapy, gentle rocking, and using a TENS device are all examples of excellent comfort measures that you can perform on your own, but in the following section, we'll focus on one that requires support from a birth partner: counterpressure.

COUNTERPRESSURE

Counterpressure involves your partner applying external pressure to your pelvis, effectively reducing the tension in the uterine ligaments and alleviating pain.

There's a misconception that applying counterpressure can reduce space in the pelvis, complicating labor. However, it's important to note that if counterpressure helps you relax during contractions, it can support your labor progress. Struggling to release tension and fighting contractions can inhibit labor progress much more than any reduction in space caused by counterpressure.

Certain counterpressure techniques increase space in the area where your baby is moving. For instance, the double hip squeeze can open the top of the pelvis, making it a preferred choice when your baby is higher in your pelvis. On the other hand, the pelvis press technique tends to open the lower part of the pelvis, which can be more suitable as your baby descends into the pelvis.

There are several counterpressure techniques you can use during your labor. I recommend practicing these during pregnancy to get a feel for where to place your hands and which positions work best for each technique.

DOUBLE HIP SQUEEZE

One of the most common counterpressure techniques is the double hip squeeze. Since everyone is unique, the exact placement of pressure may vary slightly, so you must communicate with your partner about your personal preferences.

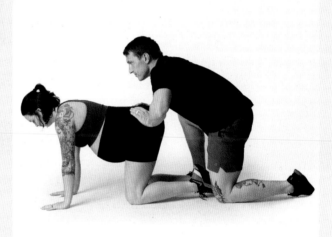

1 Find a position in which your hips are available for your partner to apply pressure. This is commonly a forward-leaning position, such as leaning on a countertop or all fours.

2 Next, your partner will feel for the bony bump of the femur head and then the indentation right above this landmark. This is usually around the widest part of your hips.

3 Your partner will place the heel of their palm into this indentation, orientating their fingertips diagonally toward the spine.

4 Your partner will apply pressure, squeezing your hips up and in toward the spine. Adjust the direction of pressure based on your personal preference.

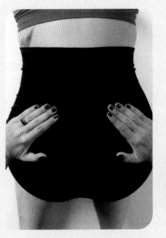
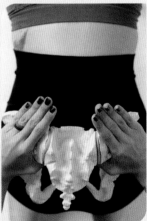

DOUBLE HIP SQUEEZE, CONT.

Variation 1: With Knees

Your partner can also apply this counterpressure technique with their knees/shins.

1 Start in an all-fours position.

2 Your partner will straddle you with their inner leg aligned with your hips.

3 Your partner will then squeeze their legs together to apply pressure to your hips.

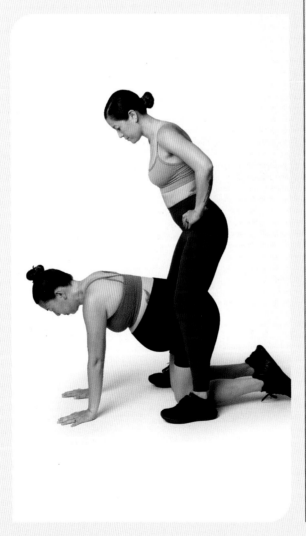

Variation 2: With Fabric (Your Partner)

Your partner can also apply counterpressure with a long piece of fabric, which can be helpful if your partner is fatigued or you want to rest in a seated or side-lying position.

1 Find a comfortable laboring position.

2 Route the fabric around your hips so the fabric is situated below your belly but across the widest part of your hips.

3 Cross the two free-running ends across the back of your hips. Do not tie a knot in the fabric.

4 Your partner will pull on each free-running end to tighten the fabric across the hips.

Variation 3: With Fabric (You)

You can apply counterpressure yourself. Try using the fabric with a wooden spoon. This variation can be helpful when you are driving to the hospital or in other situations where your partner cannot physically apply counterpressure.

1 Tie the fabric around your hips but below your belly. The knot should be oriented over the side of your hip.

2 Insert a wooden spoon, or similar stick-like object, into the knot.

3 Twist the wooden spoon to tighten the fabric.

PELVIC PRESS

The pelvic press applies pressure to the top of the hip crest and may increase the space in the bottom of the pelvis, and you can sometimes feel that the bottom of your pelvis is opening as your partner applies this pressure. This technique may be preferred as your baby moves lower in the pelvis.

1 Your partner will place their hands so the palm is cut in half by the hip crest, with fingertips oriented toward the front.

2 Apply gentle pressure directly inward. It is essential to communicate with your partner about the amount of pressure, as it is easy to apply too much pressure with this technique.

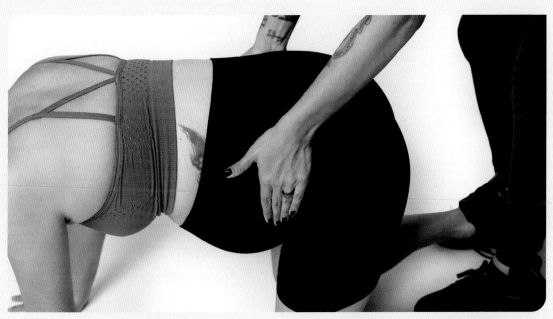

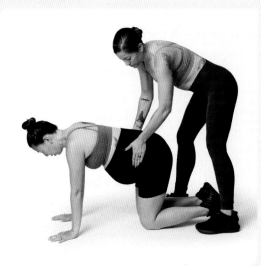

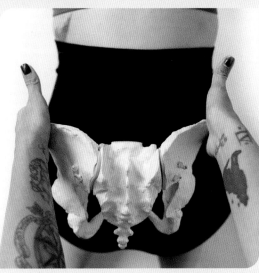

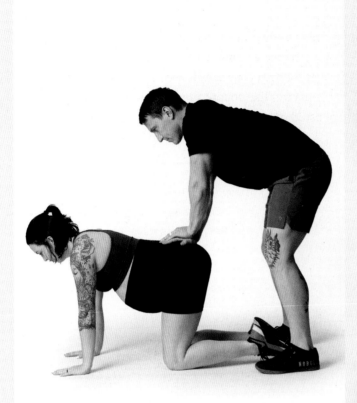

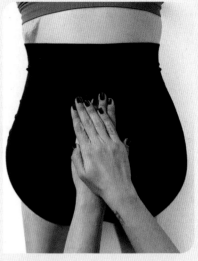

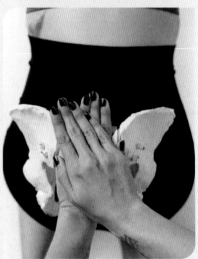

SACRAL COUNTERPRESSURE

Sacral counterpressure involves applying pressure to the sacral area, which is the back of the pelvis. The sacrum becomes more noticeable as it naturally protrudes outward when your baby descends into your pelvis. This technique can be beneficial if you have back pain with your contractions and it can be done in almost any labor position.

1 Your partner will place their hands so the palm is cut in half by the hip crest, with fingertips oriented toward the front.

2 Apply gentle pressure directly inward. It is essential to communicate with your partner about the amount of pressure, as it is easy to apply too much pressure with this technique.

KEY TAKEAWAYS

You can navigate your labor more comfortably by opening up space in your pelvis and relieving tension. During labor, you can create more space in your pelvis by adopting positions that specifically target the area your baby is trying to move through, while integrating labor comfort measures like counterpressure can help relieve tension. I hope this chapter has boosted your confidence in knowing how to manage your actual birth experience! Let's move on to the early postpartum period.

PART 4

POSTPARTUM

FINALLY! YOU'RE POSTPARTUM. Your body might feel like you just finished the hardest workout of your life, with hormones going haywire, and you're wearing a diaper to match your new baby. There is a lot going on. And, speaking of your baby, did you know that in these early weeks, they have no concept that they're a separate individual? To them, it's like you and they are one and the same, which is why they can't get enough of being in your arms all the time. It's fascinating how that strong bond works!

Motherhood is amazing, and I'm excited for you as you embark on this adventure or start a new chapter in your motherhood journey. It's difficult to fully convey how profound and transformative this journey can be in the days, weeks, and months after your baby's arrival.

In this part of the book, I'll share how to handle these early weeks. The early postpartum period is too short to rush back to the gym, yet too long to do absolutely nothing. We'll explore some gentle movements you can incorporate in these early days to support your healing without pushing yourself too hard, both physically and mentally. You've already learned many of these movements and the physiology behind them in earlier chapters, so this section will build on what you have been practicing.

NINE
EARLY POST-PARTUM (0–6 WEEKS)

WELCOME TO EARLY POSTPARTUM, which typically starts right after giving birth and extends to about 4 to 6 weeks postpartum, though it may be longer depending on your birth, such as if you had a C-section or postpartum hemorrhage. It's important to be patient with yourself, as healing may take more time than expected.

Prioritizing rest is crucial. You might feel great, but remember that inside your uterus, there's a wound the size of a dinner plate that needs to heal. If you had a vaginal birth or pushed for an extended period, your pelvic floor requires time to recover. And if you had a C-section, you underwent major abdominal surgery, making rest and recovery even more essential.

If you take the time to allow your body the opportunity to heal this first month, you will set yourself up better for your return to fitness. If you rush, you may cause more issues that you then need to overcome, in addition to the normal healing required after birth.

5-5-5: EARLY POSTPARTUM REST

During the first 2 weeks postpartum, rest is absolutely essential for starting your recovery journey. Just like if you had an ankle injury and started running too soon before it fully healed, it can lead to another injury or prolong the healing process; the same applies in the early postpartum period. I understand that it can be tough to sit around and do "nothing," especially if you're eager to get back to feeling like yourself.

You can rest primarily in bed for the first 5 days, then spend most of your time on the bed for the next 5 days, and, finally, minimize time on your feet for the last 5 days. This approach supports the initial healing of your tissues and placental wound.

However, you're not confined to bed for the entire 15 days. You can incorporate gentle movements to reconnect with your core and pelvic floor, beginning as early as the day you gave birth. This gradual approach promotes healing and rehabilitation while respecting your body's needs.

BREATHING EXERCISES

The first core exercises you can do postpartum are breathing exercises. While it may not appear like a typical core exercise, it's important to redefine what constitutes a core exercise. The core's fundamental function is stabilization—you want your core to maintain its position while the rest of your body moves. Diaphragmatic breathing serves as the cornerstone for core stabilization.

When doing breathing exercises, you can begin to sense your abdominal muscles, back muscles, and pelvic floor muscles not only moving, but also moving in coordination with one another, which is a second essential aspect of core stabilization. When you inhale, you'll notice your core and pelvic floor muscles lengthening and stretching, and when you exhale, these same muscles will shorten and contract. These breathing exercises are the foundation for reconnecting with and strengthening your core after birth.

BACK EXPANSION

While you're doing the breathing exercises, you can incorporate back expansion movements to release common areas of tension in the early postpartum. Some reasons for discomfort in the postpartum, such as pelvic heaviness, can relate to tension in the back half of your pelvic floor, so these back expansion exercises may provide a ton of relief in these targeted areas.

SUPINE OR RECLINED BREATHING EXERCISE

You can start the supine or reclined breathing exercise almost immediately after giving birth. You might find it comfortable to lie flat on your back, or you can choose a more reclined position by using some pillows for support. During the exercise, focus on feeling your back expand into your bed as you inhale, and then relax with exhales.

If you're experiencing pelvic floor discomfort, try elevating your hips by placing a pillow under them. The elevated hip position creates an anti-gravity effect that can help alleviate tension in the pelvic floor.

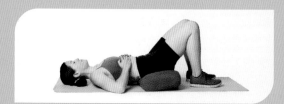

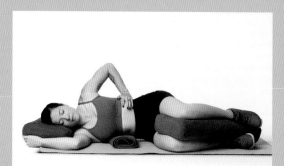

SIDE-LYING BREATHING EXERCISE

For the side-lying position, you can place a pillow or a rolled-up towel in the gap between your hip and rib cage and place a pillow between your legs. When you inhale, you'll feel your side push into the bed and your hand; exhale to relax or gently contract.

Following these breathing exercises, you can progress to more upright positions, including table-top, seated, and standing positions.

BREATHING EXERCISE

If you've had a C-section, it's important to note that this child's pose position may not be accessible due to your incision, but a more upright position, such as seated or all fours, may feel more comfortable. Eventually, you can work your way up to more upright positions, such as standing, as described in chapter 7 on page 125. In all these back expansion exercises, the focus is on rounding your back to release tension with each exhalation.

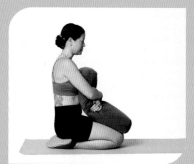

1 Hold a pillow and gently curl your body around it.

2 Inhale to expand your back.

3 Exhale to curl deeper by drawing your rib cage and pelvis closer together.

4 Repeat for 5 to 10 breaths.

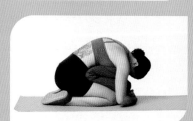

MOBILITY

If you stay in one position for prolonged periods of time, you will probably feel stiff or sore. Mobility exercises can relieve discomfort, but be careful not to overdo it and impede your healing.

THORACIC MOBILITY

The upper spine has three movements: arch and round, side bend, and rotate. Thoracic mobility exercises can provide a ton of relief, especially if your back feels stiff and sore.

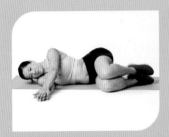
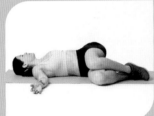

OPEN THE BOOK: SUPINE THORACIC ROTATION

One of the initial thoracic mobility exercises that can be performed in bed is the exercise called "open the book." Simply lie on your back and gently rotate your spine.

SEATED OR ALL FOURS

As you progress, you can move to a more upright position, like a seated or kneeling posture, for flexion, extension, lateral side bending, and rotation.

1 Begin by arching your back to look up toward the ceiling. This will stretch the front side of your body.

2 Round your back to tuck your chin. This will stretch the back side of your body.

3 Repeat this cycle for 5 to 10 repetitions.

4 Then reach each arm overhead and lean toward the opposite side to feel a stretch in your side.

5 You can either hold this position or move in and out 5 to 10 times.

6 Rotate your chest in one direction and then twist it toward the opposite direction.

7 If you're in a kneeling position, you can choose to thread one arm underneath the other for a deeper twist.

8 Repeat 5 to 10 times on each side.

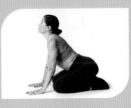
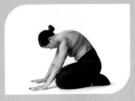
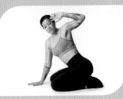
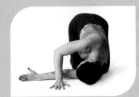

CHEST MOBILITY

The next area of focus is the chest. While holding your baby, you might notice that your shoulders tend to round forward, making your chest muscles tense. By working on chest mobility and opening up this area, you can alleviate a significant amount of discomfort and potentially find relief from any associated back pain.

FLOOR OR WALL ANGELS

1 Starting in a supine position, bring your arms out to the sides, bending your elbows at a 90-degree angle. Imagine you're trying to create a "goal post" shape with your arms.

2 Slowly reach the hands overhead while keeping your rib cage down. This motion will create a stretch in your chest as your arms move overhead.

3 Repeat this 5 to 10 times.

You can do the same movement in an upright position by progressing to wall angels. For wall angels, lean back against a wall in a seated or standing position as you reach your arms overhead.

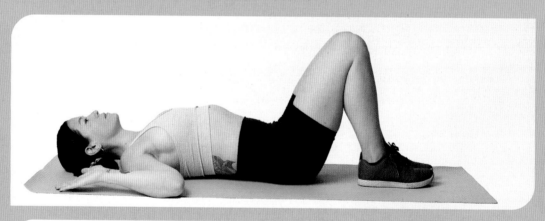

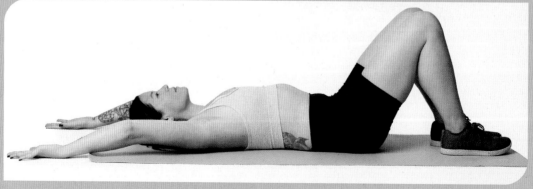

HIP MOBILITY

The final mobility focus is the hips. You can also incorporate any of the pelvic floor exercises from chapter 7 in these early days to help release tension in the pelvic floor and hips.

During the early postpartum period, you may find yourself in one position for extended periods, especially if you're following the recommendation to rest and stay mostly in bed. Gentle mobility exercises that focus on your thoracic spine, chest, and hips can help alleviate tension in these commonly affected areas to keep you comfortable as you heal postpartum.

SUPINE FIGURE FOUR

1 Start in a supine position and cross one ankle over the opposite knee, forming a figure four shape with your legs.

2 Hold this position to feel the stretch in your hip, or gently press against the lifted knee to intensify the stretch.

3 Gradually allow the lifted foot to fall toward the floor while rotating your upper body and hips.

4 Maintain this position for 5 to 10 breaths, then switch sides.

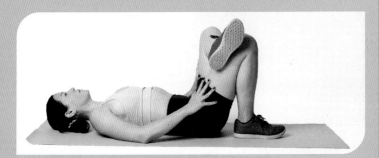

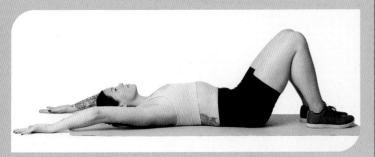

ALL-FOURS HIP SHIFT

By now, you should be familiar with hip shifts, especially the all-fours hip shift. This movement can be added to your early postpartum routine to release tension in the pelvic floor and hips.

1 Start in a tabletop position, and place a pillow or yoga block under one knee.

2 Shift your weight toward the elevated hip to feel more of a stretch in the elevated hip.

3 Stay here for 5 to 10 breaths.

4 You have the option to add in pelvic tilts in this shifted position. If so, perform 5 to 10 pelvic tilts.

GENTLE CORE EXERCISES

The key to these core exercises is maintaining your torso position as your arms or legs move, while coordinating your breathing. Reestablishing this breath-to-movement coordination is necessary to build off for your return to fitness.

This core stabilization series challenges the core in three different positions. Start in a supine position, then a side plank position, and finish in a tabletop position.

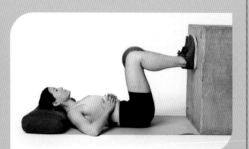

90/90 HIP LIFT

In the 90/90 hip lift, focus on activating the hamstrings and glutes to lift your hips off the floor. Although your arms and legs are not moving yet, you are beginning to incorporate muscular activation of the legs in coordination with your breathing.

1 Start in the supine position with your legs in a 90-degree angle and your feet pressing into the wall.

2 Focus on driving your heels downward without moving your feet. This will increase the activation of your hamstrings.

3 Inhale to feel your back push into the ground.

4 Exhale to lift your hips off the ground.

5 Lower the hips to the floor and repeat 5 to 10 times.

DEADBUG ARMS ONLY

Next, you can progress the 90/90 hip lift by incorporating arm movements. As you move your arm overhead, focus on keeping your rib cage down. You can even think about or actively pull the rib cage and pelvis closer together on the front side of the body as you lift the arm overhead.

1 Repeat steps 1 to 3 of the previous exercise.

2 Exhale to extend one arm overhead as you lift the hips off the ground, keeping the rib cage down and avoid arching your back.

3 Return to the starting position and repeat 5 to 10 times.

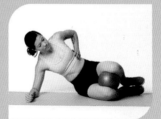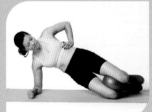

SIDE-LYING HIP ABDUCTION

This position challenges the side of your body and obliques to maintain the alignment of the rib cage and pelvis as you move. Think of this movement as doing a sideways glute bridge: the hips will move forward to extend, not lift directly upward to the ceiling. See page 57 for a detailed breakdown of this exercise.

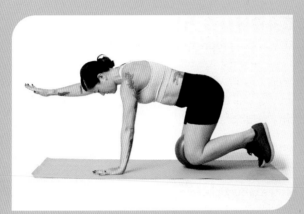

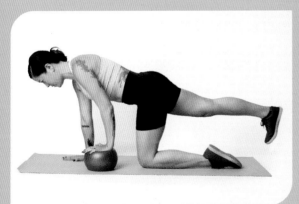

BIRD DOG ARMS, THEN LEGS ONLY

Next, you can progress to adding in the movement of one arm or leg in the tabletop position.

1 Start in a tabletop position.

2 Exhale to extend one arm forward without arching the back.

3 Inhale to lower the arm to the floor.

4 Repeat 5 to 10 times with each arm.

5 Progress to moving just one leg at a time; exhale to extend one leg backward, keeping the toe fairly close to the ground.

6 Avoid arching your back as you extend the leg backward.

7 Inhale to return to the starting position.

8 Repeat 5 to 10 times with each leg.

TABLETOP KNEE LIFT

In this position, focus on maintaining the position of the torso without arching your back. Similar to the 90/90 hip lift, try to maintain the position as you add a little movement.

1 Start in a tabletop position.

2 Exhale to hover the knees off the floor.

3 Inhale to lower.

4 Repeat 5 to 10 times.

WALKING

You can gradually introduce short walks and increase your overall movement, both indoors and outdoors. These walks can be relatively short, ranging from 5 to 20 minutes in duration.

While going for these walks, monitor your bleeding levels before and after each walk. If you notice that your bleeding increases after the walk, it may indicate that you've exerted too much effort, and you may want to prioritize rest for the remainder of the day. However, if your bleeding remains the same or decreases, you can continue to gradually progress your activity levels.

SAMPLE EARLY POSTPARTUM MOVEMENT GUIDE

In the early postpartum period, you want to start incorporating some sort of movement and rehabilitation exercises, but in a way that is manageable. You may do one or two movements a day and rest the remainder of the day, or do several movements and go for a walk.

SAMPLE EARLY POSTPARTUM MOVEMENT GUIDE

WEEK	BREATHING DRILL	MOBILITY	GENTLE CORE EXERCISES
Week 1	Supine breathing Child's pose back expansion	Supine thoracic mobility Supine chest angels	None
Week 2	Seated breathing Seated back expansion Side-lying breathing	Seated thoracic mobility Seated chest angels	None
Week 3	Tabletop breathing All fours back expansion	All-fours thoracic mobility All-fours chest mobility 90/90 side opener	90/90 hip lift Side-lying hip abduction Tabletop knee lift Short walks
Week 4+	Standing breathing Standing back expansion	Lat stretch with wall Standing chest mobility	Deadbug: arms only Side-lying hip abduction Bird dog: arms only Bird dog: legs only Short walks

You can use this very general guide to help you progress movements from week to week while incorporating movements from previous weeks. Know that this is very general—you do not need to progress on this timeline. You can move slower through this timeline, but I don't recommend progressing faster and rushing this process.

KEY TAKEAWAYS

The early postpartum period is a unique phase where it's crucial to strike a balance. It's too brief to rush back into intense workouts or gym sessions, but it's also too long to remain completely inactive. You can begin by integrating breathing exercises to learn how to engage your core and pelvic floor muscles in coordination with your breath, which lays the foundation for rebuilding core stabilization and functional movement.

Additionally, gentle mobility exercises can help you stay comfortable without hindering your healing process. Then, you can progress toward incorporating some gentle core exercises. This further enhances core stabilization and establishes a solid foundation to build from in your return to fitness.

Honoring this is the early postpartum phase, and taking it slow is crucial. Rushing through these initial weeks could impede your healing and lead to long-term issues. By being patient and intentional in the first month, you set the stage for a healthier and more robust postpartum recovery. In the long run, you'll be able to do it all without being in pain. Trust in the process and listen to your body.

CONCLUSION

HOPEFULLY, AFTER READING THIS BOOK, you have a better understanding of how important it is to exercise throughout your pregnancy, and you feel more confident approaching workouts. There is a lot of misinformation about the safety of prenatal exercise for both you and your baby, so it's understandable that you may have started this book wondering whether exercise was even safe to do. You should absolutely exercise throughout your pregnancy, and not doing so may be more detrimental. There is no "better safe than sorry" when it comes to prenatal fitness recommendations—not exercising can negatively affect your comfort during pregnancy, your baby's growth and development, and your preparation for birth.

Exercising enhances most of the physiological adaptations that occur during pregnancy, all of which can improve your prenatal experience and positively affect your birth. You can have a strong and pain-free pregnancy, where you feel capable and functional throughout to meet your daily demands of just being pregnant (and chasing around any other kids you have), plus prepare for your birth with pelvic opening and pelvic floor exercises. And then, your efforts during your pregnancy can hasten your recovery after birth, supporting a return to fitness that affects not only your physical health but also your mental health.

For your baby, exercising throughout your pregnancy can positively affect their brain, nervous system, and musculoskeletal development. These effects are noticed in your baby's first year of life through their improved motor and cognitive skills. And then these effects can continue to be seen as they reach elementary school years and beyond. Your dedication to your workouts is worth the effort just for this reason alone.

I hope you can continue to use this book as a reference to support your entire pregnancy and birth journey, and I am grateful that you chose me to support you during this awe-inspiring chapter of your life. Thank you!

—Gina

REFERENCES

CHAPTER 1

1. Wadhwa, Yogyata, Ahmad H. Alghadir, and Zaheen A. Iqbal. "Effect of Antenatal Exercises, Including Yoga, on the Course of Labor, Delivery and Pregnancy: A Retrospective Study." *International Journal of Environmental Research and Public Health* 17, no. 15 (2020): 5274.

2. Davenport, Margie H., Stephanie-May Ruchat, Veronica J. Poitras, Alejandra Jaramillo Garcia, Casey E. Gray, Nick Barrowman, Rachel J. Skow et al. "Prenatal Exercise for the Prevention of Gestational Diabetes Mellitus and Hypertensive Disorders of Pregnancy: A Systematic Review and Meta-Analysis." *British Journal of Sports Medicine* 52, no. 21 (2018): 1367-1375.

3. Vargas-Terrones, Marina, Ruben Barakat, Belen Santacruz, Irene Fernandez-Buhigas, and Michelle F. Mottola. "Physical Exercise Programme During Pregnancy Decreases Perinatal Depression Risk: A Randomised Controlled Trial." *British Journal of Sports Medicine* 53, no. 6 (2019): 348-353.

4. Watts, Nelson B., Neil Binkley, Charlotte D. Owens, Ayman Al-Hendy, Elizabeth E. Puscheck, Mohamad Shebley, William D. Schlaff, and James A. Simon. "Bone Mineral Density Changes Associated with Pregnancy, Lactation, and Medical Treatments in Premenopausal Women and Effects Later in Life." *Journal of Women's Health* 30, no. 10 (2021): 1416-1430.

5. Barakat, Ruben, Ignacio Refoyo, Javier Coteron, and Evelia Franco. "Exercise During Pregnancy Has a Preventative Effect on Excessive Maternal Weight Gain and Gestational Diabetes. A Randomized Controlled Trial." *Brazilian Journal of Physical Therapy* 23, no. 2 (2019): 148-155.

6. Laredo-Aguilera, José Alberto, María Gallardo-Bravo, Joseba Aingerun Rabanales-Sotos, Ana Isabel Cobo-Cuenca, and Juan Manuel Carmona-Torres. "Physical Activity Programs During Pregnancy Are Effective for the Control of Gestational Diabetes Mellitus." *International Journal of Environmental Research and Public Health* 17, no. 17 (2020): 6151.

7. Huifen, Zhao, Xie Yaping, Zhao Meijing, Huang Huibin, Liu Chunhong, Huang Fengfeng, and Zhang Yaping. "Effects of Moderate-Intensity Resistance Exercise on Blood Glucose and Pregnancy Outcome in Patients with Gestational Diabetes Mellitus: A Randomized Controlled Trial." *Journal of Diabetes and Its Complications* 36, no. 5 (2022): 108186.

8. Goossens, Nina, Hugo Massé-Alarie, Daniela Aldabe, Jonas Verbrugghe, and Lotte Janssens. "Changes in Static Balance During Pregnancy and Postpartum: A Systematic Review." *Gait & Posture* 96 (2022): 160-172.

9. Conder, Rebecca, Reza Zamani, and Mohammad Akrami. "The Biomechanics of Pregnancy: A Systematic Review." *Journal of Functional Morphology and Kinesiology* 4, no. 4 (2019): 72.

10. Quesada Salazar, Natalia. "Musculoskeletal Changes and Biomechanic Adaptations During the Three Trimesters of Pregnancy: A Systematic Review." *Pensar en Movimiento: Revista de Ciencias del Ejercicio y la Salud* 19, no. 1 (2021): 161-187.

11. Davenport, Margie H., Ashley P. McCurdy, Michelle F. Mottola, Rachel J. Skow, Victoria L. Meah, Veronica J. Poitras, Alejandra Jaramillo Garcia et al. "Impact of Prenatal Exercise on Both Prenatal and Postnatal Anxiety and Depressive Symptoms: A Systematic Review and Meta-Analysis." *British Journal of Sports Medicine* 52, no. 21 (2018): 1376-1385.

12. Kołomańska-Bogucka, Daria, and Agnieszka Irena Mazur-Bialy. "Physical Activity and the Occurrence of Postnatal Depression—A Systematic Review." *Medicina* 55, no. 9 (2019): 560.

13. Ranković, Goran, Vlada Mutavdžić, Dragan Toskić, Adem Preljević, Miodrag Kocić, Gorana Nedin-Ranković, and Nikola Damjanović. "Aerobic Capacity as an Indicator in Different Kinds of Sports." *Bosnian Journal of Basic Medical Sciences* 10, no. 1 (2010): 44.

CHAPTER 2

1. Davenport, Margie H., Victoria L. Meah, Stephanie-May Ruchat, Gregory A. Davies, Rachel J. Skow, Nick Barrowman, Kristi B. Adamo et al. "Impact of Prenatal Exercise on Neonatal and Childhood Outcomes: A Systematic Review and Meta-Analysis." *British Journal of Sports Medicine* 52, no. 21 (2018): 1386-96. https://doi.org/10.1136/bjsports-2018-099836.

2. Davenport, Margie H., Amariah J. Kathol, Michelle F. Mottola, Rachel J. Skow, Victoria L. Meah, Veronica J. Poitras, Alejandra Jaramillo Garcia et al. "Prenatal Exercise Is Not Associated with Fetal Mortality: A Systematic Review and Meta-Analysis." *British Journal of Sports Medicine* 53, no. 2 (2019): 108-115.

3. Baena-García, Laura, Marta de la Flor-Alemany, Irene Coll-Risco, Olga Roldán Reoyo, Pilar Aranda, and Virginia A. Aparicio. "A Concurrent Prenatal Exercise Program Increases Neonatal and Placental Weight and Shortens Labor: The GESTAFIT Project." *Scandinavian Journal of Medicine & Science in Sports* 33, no. 4 (2023): 465-474.

4. Collings, Paul J., Diane Farrar, Joanna Gibson, Jane West, Sally E. Barber, and John Wright. "Associations of Pregnancy Physical Activity with Maternal Cardiometabolic Health, Neonatal Delivery Outcomes and Body Composition in a Biethnic Cohort of 7305 Mother–Child Pairs: The Born in Bradford Study." *Sports Medicine* 50, no. 3 (2020): 615-628.

5. Clapp, James F., Hyungjin Kim, Brindusa Burciu, and Beth Lopez. "Beginning Regular Exercise in Early Pregnancy: Effect on Fetoplacental Growth." *American Journal of Obstetrics and Gynecology* 183, no. 6 (2000): 1484-88. https://doi.org/10.1067/mob.2000.107096.

6. Menke, Brenna R., Cathryn Duchette, Rachel A. Tinius, Alexandria Q. Wilson, Elizabeth A. Altizer, and Jill M. Maples. "Physical Activity During Pregnancy and Newborn Body Composition: A Systematic Review." *International Journal of Environmental Research and Public Health* 19, no. 12 (2022): 7127. https://doi.org/10.3390/ijerph19127127.

7. Skow, Rachel J., Margie H. Davenport, Michelle F. Mottola, Gregory A. Davies, Veronica J. Poitras, Casey E. Gray, Alejandra Jaramillo Garcia et al. "Effects of Prenatal Exercise on Fetal Heart Rate, Umbilical and Uterine Blood Flow: A Systematic Review and Meta-Analysis." *British Journal of Sports Medicine* 53, no. 2 (2019): 124-133. https://doi.org/10.1136/bjsports-2018-099822.

8. Davenport, Margie H., Stephanie-May Ruchat, Frances Sobierajski, Veronica J. Poitras, Casey E. Gray, Courtney Yoo, Rachel J. Skow et al. "Impact

of Prenatal Exercise on Maternal Harms, Labour and Delivery Outcomes: A Systematic Review and Meta-Analysis." *British Journal of Sports Medicine* 53, no. 2 (2019): 99-107. https://doi.org/10.1136/bjsports-2018-099821.

9. McMillan, Amy Gross, Linda E. May, Georgeanna Gower Gaines, Christy Isler, and Devon Kuehn. "Effects of Aerobic Exercise During Pregnancy on One-Month Infant Neuromotor Skills." *Medicine & Science in Sports & Exercise* 51, no. 8 (2019): 1671-1676.

10. de Andrade Leão, Otávio Amaral, Marlos Rodrigues Domingues, Andréa Dâmaso Bertoldi, Luiza Isnardi Cardoso Ricardo, Werner de Andrade Müller, Luciana Tornquist et al. "Effects of Regular Exercise During Pregnancy on Early Childhood Neurodevelopment: The Physical Activity for Mothers Enrolled in Longitudinal Analysis Randomized Controlled Trial." *Journal of Physical Activity and Health* 19, no. 3 (2022): 203-210.

11. Vidarsdottir, Harpa, Reynir Tomas Geirsson, Hildur Hardardottir, Unnur Valdimarsdottir, and Atli Dagbjartsson. "Obstetric and Neonatal Risks among Extremely Macrosomic Babies and Their Mothers." *American Journal of Obstetrics and Gynecology* 204, no. 5 (2011): 423.e1-423.e6. https://doi.org/10.1016/j.ajog.2010.12.036.

12. Siggelkow, W., D. Boehm, C. Skala, M. Grosslercher, M. Schmidt, and H. Koelbl. "The Influence of Macrosomia on the Duration of Labor, the Mode of Delivery and Intrapartum Complications." *Archives of Gynecology and Obstetrics* 278, no. 6 (2008): 547–553. https://doi.org/10.1007/s00404-008-0630-7.

13. Henriksen, Tore. "The Macrosomic Fetus: A Challenge in Current Obstetrics." *Acta Obstetricia et Gynecologica Scandinavica* 87 no. 2 (2008): 134–145. https://doi.org/10.1080/00016340801899289.

14. Boulet, Sheree L., Greg R. Alexander, Hamisu M. Salihu, and MaryAnn Pass. "Macrosomic Births in the United States: Determinants, Outcomes, and Proposed Grades of Risk." *American Journal of Obstetrics and Gynecology* 188 no. 5 (2003): 1372-1378. https://doi.org/10.1067/mob.2003.302.

15. Chawanpaiboon, Saifon, Vitaya Titapant, and Julaporn Pooliam. "Maternal Complications and Risk Factors Associated with Assisted Vaginal Delivery." *BMC Pregnancy and Childbirth* 23, no. 1 (2023): 756. https://doi.org/10.1186/s12884-023-06080-9.

16. Jolly, Matthew C., Neil J. Sebire, John P. Harris, Lesley Regan, and Stephen Robinson. "Risk Factors for Macrosomia and Its Clinical Consequences: A Study of 350,311 Pregnancies." *European Journal of Obstetrics & Gynecology and Reproductive Biology* 111, no. 1 (2003): 9-14.

CHAPTER 3

1. Barakat, Rubén, Dingfeng Zhang, Cristina Silva-José, Miguel Sánchez-Polán, Evelia Franco, and Michelle F. Mottola. "The Influence of Physical Activity during Pregnancy on Miscarriage—Systematic Review and Meta-Analysis." *Journal of Clinical Medicine* 12, no. 16 (2023): 5393.

2. Davenport, Margie H., Amariah J. Kathol, Michelle F. Mottola, Rachel J. Skow, Victoria L. Meah, Veronica J. Poitras, Alejandra Jaramillo Garcia et al. "Prenatal Exercise Is Not Associated with Fetal Mortality: A Systematic Review and Meta-Analysis." *British Journal of Sports Medicine* 53, no. 2 (2019): 108-115.

3. Meah, Victoria L., Gregory A. Davies, and Margie H. Davenport. "Why Can't I Exercise During Pregnancy? Time to Revisit Medical 'Absolute' and 'Relative' Contraindications: Systematic Review of Evidence of Harm and a Call to Action." *British Journal of Sports Medicine* 54, no. 23 (2020): 1395-1404.

4. Sundgot-Borgen, Jorunn, Christine Sundgot-Borgen, Grethe Myklebust, Nina Sølvberg, and Monica Klungland Torstveit. "Elite Athletes Get Pregnant, Have Healthy Babies and Return to Sport Early Postpartum." *BMJ Open Sport & Exercise Medicine* 5, no. 1 (2019): e000652.

5. Wowdzia, Jenna B., Tara-Leigh McHugh, Jane Thornton, Allison Sivak, Michelle F. Mottola, and Margie H. Davenport. "Elite Athletes and Pregnancy Outcomes: A Systematic Review and Meta-Analysis." *Medicine & Science in Sports & Exercise* 53, no. 3 (2021): 534-542.

6. Tinloy, Jennifer, Cynthia H. Chuang, Junjia Zhu, Jaimey Pauli, Jennifer L. Kraschnewski, and Kristen H. Kjerulff. "Exercise During Pregnancy and Risk of Late Preterm Birth, Cesarean Delivery, and Hospitalizations." *Women's Health Issues* 24, no. 1 (2014): e99-e104.

7. Nuss, Emily E., and Anthony C. Sciscione. "Activity Restriction and Preterm Birth Prevention." *Current Opinion in Obstetrics and Gynecology* 34, no. 2 (2022): 77-81.

8. Matenchuk, Brittany, Rshmi Khurana, Chenxi Cai, Normand G. Boulé, Linda Slater, and Margie H. Davenport. "Prenatal Bed Rest in Developed and Developing Regions: A Systematic Review and Meta-Analysis." *Canadian Medical Association Open Access Journal* 7, no. 3 (2019): E435-E445.

9. Walsh, Colin A. "Maternal Activity Restriction to Reduce Preterm Birth: Time to Put This Fallacy to Bed." *Australian and New Zealand Journal of Obstetrics and Gynaecology* 60, no. 5 (2020): 813-815.

10. Ravanelli, Nicholas, William Casasola, Timothy English, Kate M. Edwards, and Ollie Jay. "Heat Stress and Fetal Risk. Environmental Limits for Exercise and Passive Heat Stress During Pregnancy: A Systematic Review with Best Evidence Synthesis." *British Journal of Sports Medicine* 53, no. 13 (2019): 799-805.

11. Smallcombe, James W., Agalyaa Puhenthirar, William Casasola, Daniela S. Inoue, Georgia K. Chaseling, Nicholas Ravanelli, Kate M. Edwards, and Ollie Jay. "Thermoregulation During Pregnancy: A Controlled Trial Investigating the Risk of Maternal Hyperthermia During Exercise in the Heat." *Sports Medicine (Auckland)* 51, no. 12 (2021): 2655-64. https://doi.org/10.1007/s40279-021-01504-y.

12. Davenport, Margie H., Courtney Yoo, Michelle F. Mottola, Veronica J. Poitras, Alejandra Jaramillo Garcia, Casey E. Gray, Nick Barrowman et al. "Effects of Prenatal Exercise on Incidence of Congenital Anomalies and Hyperthermia: A Systematic Review and Meta-Analysis." *British Journal of Sports Medicine* 53, no. 2 (2019): 116-123.

13. Davenport, Margie H., Stephanie-May Ruchat, Frances Sobierajski, Veronica J. Poitras, Casey E. Gray, Courtney Yoo, Rachel J. Skow et al. "Impact of Prenatal Exercise on Maternal Harms, Labour and Delivery Outcomes: A Systematic Review and Meta-Analysis." *British Journal of Sports Medicine* 53, no. 2 (2019): 99-107. https://doi.org/10.1136/bjsports-2018-099821.

14. Mottola, Michelle F., Taniya S. Nagpal, Roberta Bgeginski, Margie H. Davenport, Veronica J. Poitras, Casey E. Gray, Gregory A. Davies, et al. "Is Supine Exercise Associated with Adverse Maternal and Fetal Outcomes? A Systematic Review." *British Journal of Sports Medicine* 53, no. 2 (2019): 82-89. https://doi.org/10.1136/bjsports-2018-099919.

15. Jeffreys R. M., Stepanchak W., Lopez B., Hardis, J., Clapp, J.F. "Uterine Blood Flow During Supine Rest and Exercise after 28 Weeks of Gestation." *British Journal of Obstetrics and Gynaecology* 113 (2006): 1239-1247. doi:10.1111/j.1471-0528.2006.01056.x

16. Nesler C. L., Hassett S. L., Cary S., and Brooke J. "Effects of Supine Exercise on Fetal Heart Rate in the Second and Third Trimesters." *American Journal of Perinatology Reports* 5 (1988): 159-163. doi:10.1055/s-2007-999677

17. Bø, Kari, Raul Artal, Ruben Barakat, Wendy J. Brown, Gregory A. L. Davies, Michael Dooley, Kelly R. Evenson, et al. "Exercise and Pregnancy in Recreational and Elite Athletes: 2016/2017 Evidence Summary from the IOC Expert Group Meeting, Lausanne. Part 5. Recommendations for Health Professionals and Active Women." *British Journal of Sports Medicine* 52 no. 17 (2018): 1080-1085. https://doi.org/10.1136/bjsports-2018-099351.

CHAPTER 4

1. Franklin, Mary E., and Teresa Conner-Kerr. "An Analysis of Posture and Back Pain in the First and Third Trimesters of Pregnancy." *Journal of Orthopaedic & Sports Physical Therapy* 28, no. 3 (1998): 133-138.

2. Clapp, James F., Hyungjin Kim, Brindusa Burciu, and Beth Lopez. "Beginning Regular Exercise in Early Pregnancy: Effect on Fetoplacental Growth." *American Journal of Obstetrics and Gynecology* 183, no. 6 (2000): 1484-1488. https://doi.org/10.1067/mob.2000.107096.

3. Sperstad, Jorun Bakken, Merete Kolberg Tennfjord, Gunvor Hilde, Marie Ellström-Engh, and Kari Bø. "Diastasis Recti Abdominis During Pregnancy and 12 Months after Childbirth: Prevalence, Risk Factors and Report of Lumbopelvic Pain." *British Journal of Sports Medicine* 50, no. 17 (2016): 1092-1096.

4. Lee, Diane, and Paul W. Hodges. "Behavior of the Linea Alba During a Curl-Up Task in Diastasis Rectus Abdominis: An Observational Study." *Journal of Orthopaedic & Sports Physical Therapy* 46, no. 7 (2016): 580-589.

5. Lee, Diane G., Linda-Joy Lee, and L. McLaughlin. "Stability, Continence and Breathing: The Role of Fascia Following Pregnancy and Delivery." *Journal of Bodywork and Movement Therapies* 12, no. 4 (2008): 333-348.

6. Kim, Seungmin, Jhosedyn Carolaym Salazar Fajardo, and BumChul Yoon. "Activation of Anterolateral Abdominal Muscles During Sling Bridge Exercises: Comparison of Different Pelvic Positions." *Journal of Sport Rehabilitation* 1, no. 4 (2023): 376-384.

7. Myers, Thomas W. *Anatomy Trains: Myofascial Meridians for Manual and Movement Therapists.* Elsevier Health Sciences, 2009.

8. Vleeming, Andry, and Mark Schuenke. "Form and Force Closure of the Sacroiliac Joints." *PM&R* 11 (2019): S24-S31.

9. Lee, Diane. "Instability of the Sacroiliac Joint and the Consequences to Gait." *Journal of Manual & Manipulative Therapy* 4, no. 1 (1996): 22-29.

CHAPTER 5

1. Aldabe, Daniela, Stephan Milosavljevic, and Melanie Dawn Bussey. "Is Pregnancy Related Pelvic Girdle Pain Associated with Altered Kinematic, Kinetic and Motor Control of the Pelvis? A Systematic Review." *European Spine Journal* 21 (2012): 1777-1787.

2. Stuge, Britt, Even Lærum, Gitle Kirkesola, and Nina Vøllestad. "The Efficacy of a Treatment Program Focusing on Specific Stabilizing Exercises for Pelvic Girdle Pain after Pregnancy: A Randomized Controlled Trial." *Spine Journal* (2004): 351-359.

3. Morino, Saori, Mika Ishihara, Fumiko Umezaki, Hiroko Hatanaka, Mamoru Yamashita, and Tomoki Aoyama. "Pelvic Alignment Changes During the Perinatal Period." *PloS one* 14, no. 10 (2019): e0223776.

4. Franklin, Mary E., and Teresa Conner-Kerr. "An Analysis of Posture and Back Pain in the First and Third Trimesters of Pregnancy." *Journal of Orthopaedic & Sports Physical Therapy* 28, no. 3 (1998): 133-138.

5. Christensen, Lene, Marit B. Veierød, Nina K. Vølles- tad, Vidar E. Jakobsen, Britt Stuge, Jan Cabri, and Hilde Stendal Robinson. "Kinematic and Spatio- temporal Gait Characteristics in Pregnant Women with Pelvic Girdle Pain, Asymptomatic Pregnant and Non-Pregnant Women." *Clinical Biomechanics* 68 (2019): 45-52.

6. Foti, Theresa, Jon R. Davids, and Anita Bagley. "A Bio- mechanical Analysis of Gait During Pregnancy." *JBJS* 82, no. 5 (2000): 625.

CHAPTER 6

1. Borg-Stein, Joanne, Sheila A. Dugan, and Jane Gruber. "Musculoskeletal Aspects of Pregnancy." *American Journal of Physical Medicine & Rehabilitation* 84, no. 3 (2005): 180-192.

2. Betsch, Marcel, Regina Wehrle, Larissa Dor, Walter Rapp, Pascal Jungbluth, Mohssen Hakimi, and Michael Wild. "Spinal Posture and Pelvic Position During Preg- nancy: A Prospective Rasterstereographic Pilot Study." *European Spine Journal* 24, no. 6 (2015): 1282-1288. https://doi.org/10.1007/s00586-014-3521-6.

3. Yoo, Hyunju, Doochul Shin, and Changho Song. "Changes in the Spinal Curvature, Degree of Pain, Bal- ance Ability, and Gait Ability According to Pregnancy Period in Pregnant and Nonpregnant Women." *Journal of Physical Therapy Science* 27, no. 1 (2015): 279-284.

4. Morrison, Pamela. "Musculoskeletal Conditions Related to Pelvic Floor Muscle Overactivity." *The Overactive Pelvic Floor* (2016): 91-111.

5. Skalski, Matthew R., George R. Matcuk, Dakshesh B. Patel, Anderanik Tomasian, Eric A. White, and Jordan S. Gross. "Imaging Coccygeal Trauma and Coccydy- nia." *Radiographics* 40, no. 4 (2020): 1090-1106.

6. Garg, Bhavuk, and Kaustubh Ahuja. "Coccydynia: A Comprehensive Review on Etiology, Radiological

Features and Management Options." *Journal of Clini- cal Orthopaedics and Trauma* 12, no. 1 (2021): 123-129.

7. Conder, Rebecca, Reza Zamani, and Mohammad Akrami. "The Biomechanics of Pregnancy: A System- atic Review." *Journal of Functional Morphology and Kinesiology* 4, no. 4 (2019): 72.

8. Manyozo, Steven. "Low Back Pain During Pregnancy: Prevalence, Risk Factors and Association with Daily Activities among Pregnant Women in Urban Blan- tyre, Malawi." *Malawi Medical Journal* 31, no. 1 (2019): 71-76.

9. Papi, Enrica, Anthony M. J. Bull, and Alison H. McGregor. "Alteration of Movement Patterns in Low Back Pain Assessed by Statistical Parametric Map- ping." *Journal of Biomechanics* 100 (2020): 109597.

10. Bontrup, Carolin, William R. Taylor, Michael Fliesser, Rosa Visscher, Tamara Green, Pia-Maria Wippert, and Roland Zemp. "Low Back Pain and Its Relation- ship with Sitting Behaviour among Sedentary Office Workers." *Applied Ergonomics* 81 (2019): 102894.

11. Christensen, Lene, Marit B. Veierød, Nina K. Vølles- tad, Vidar E. Jakobsen, Britt Stuge, Jan Cabri, and Hilde Stendal Robinson. "Kinematic and Spatio- temporal Gait Characteristics in Pregnant Women with Pelvic Girdle Pain, Asymptomatic Pregnant and Non-Pregnant Women." *Clinical Biomechanics* 68 (2019): 45-52.

12. Davenport, Margie H., Andree-Anne Marchand, Michelle F. Mottola, Veronica J. Poitras, Casey E. Gray, Alejandra Jaramillo Garcia, Nick Barrowman et al. "Exercise for the Prevention and Treatment of Low Back, Pelvic Girdle and Lumbopelvic Pain During Pregnancy: A Systematic Review and Meta-Analysis." *British Journal of Sports Medicine* 53, no. 2 (2019): 90-98.

13. Quintero Rodriguez, Carolina, and Olga Troynikov. "The Effect of Maternity Support Garments on

Alleviation of Pains and Discomforts During Pregnancy: A Systematic Review." *Journal of Pregnancy* 2019 (2019).

14. ACOG. *Gestational Hypertension and Preeclampsia*, June 2020. https://www.acog.org/clinical/clinical-guidance/practice-bulletin/articles/2020/06/gestational-hypertension-and-preeclampsia.

15. August, Phyllis, and Baha M. Sibai. "Preeclampsia: Clinical Features and Diagnosis." *UpToDate* Accessed December 22 (2017).

16. LoMauro, Antonella, and Andrea Aliverti. "Respiratory Physiology in Pregnancy and Assessment of Pulmonary Function." *Best Practice & Research Clinical Obstetrics & Gynaecology* (2022).

17. Bacaro, Valeria, Fee Benz, Andrea Pappaccogli, Paola De Bartolo, Anna F. Johann, Laura Palagini, Caterina Lombardo, Bernd Feige, Dieter Riemann, and Chiara Baglioni. "Interventions for Sleep Problems During Pregnancy: A Systematic Review." *Sleep Medicine Reviews* 50 (2020): 101234.

18. Richter, J. E. "The Management of Heartburn in Pregnancy." *Alimentary Pharmacology & Therapeutics* 22, no. 9 (2005): 749-757.

CHAPTER 7

1. Iversen, Johanne Kolvik, Birgitte Heiberg Kahrs, and Torbjørn Moe Eggebø. "There Are 4, Not 7, Cardinal Movements in Labor." *American Journal of Obstetrics & Gynecology MFM* 3, no. 6 (2021): 100436.

2. Siccardi, Marco A., Onyebuchi Imonugo, and Cristina Valle. "Anatomy, Abdomen and Pelvis, Pelvic Inlet." In *StatPearls* [*Internet*] . StatPearls Publishing, 2018. .

3. Siccardi, Marco, Cristina Valle, and Fiorenza Di Matteo. "Dynamic External Pelvimetry Test in Third Trimester Pregnant Women: Shifting Positions Affect Pelvic Biomechanics and Create More Room in Obstetric Diameters." *Cureus* 13, no. 3 (2021).

4. Drerup, Burkhard, and Eberhard Hierholzer. "Movement of the Human Pelvis and Displacement of Related Anatomical Landmarks on the Body Surface." *Journal of Biomechanics* 20, no. 10 (1987): 971-977.

5. Reitter, Anke, Betty-Anne Daviss, Andrew Bisits, Astrid Schollenberger, Thomas Vogl, Eva Herrmann, Frank Louwen, and Stephan Zangos. "Does Pregnancy and/or Shifting Positions Create More Room in a Woman's Pelvis?" *American Journal of Obstetrics and Gynecology* 211, no. 6 (2014): 662-e1.

6. McEvoy, Austin, and Maggie Tetrokalashvili. "Anatomy, Abdomen and Pelvis, Female Pelvic Cavity." In *StatPearls* [*Internet*]. StatPearls Publishing, 2019.

7. Flusberg, Milana, Mariya Kobi, Simin Bahrami, Phyllis Glanc, Suzanne Palmer, Victoria Chernyak, Devaraju Kanmaniraja, and Rania Farouk El Sayed. "Multimodality Imaging of Pelvic Floor Anatomy." *Abdominal Radiology* 46 (2021): 1302-1311.

8. Raizada, Varuna, and Ravinder K. Mittal. "Pelvic Floor Anatomy and Applied Physiology." *Gastroenterology Clinics of North America* 37, no. 3 (2008): 493-509.

9. Silva, M. E. T., D. A. Oliveira, T. H. Roza, S. Brandao, M. P. L. Parente, T. Mascarenhas, and RM Natal Jorge. "Study on the Influence of the Fetus Head Molding on the Biomechanical Behavior of the Pelvic Floor Muscles, During Vaginal Delivery." *Journal of Biomechanics* 48, no. 9 (2015): 1600-1605.

10. Oleksy, Łukasz, Anna Mika, Renata Kielnar, Joanna Grzegorczyk, Anna Marchewka, and Artur Stolarczyk. "The Influence of Pelvis Reposition Exercises on Pelvic Floor Muscles Asymmetry: A Randomized Prospective Study." *Medicine* 98, no. 2 (2019).

11. Aljuraifani, Rafeef, Ryan E. Stafford, Leanne M. Hall, Wolbert Van den Hoorn, and Paul W. Hodges. "Task-Specific Differences in Respiration-Related Activation of Deep and Superficial Pelvic Floor Muscles." *Journal of Applied Physiology* 126, no. 5 (2019): 1343-1351.

12. Eggleton, Julie S., and Bruno Cunha. "Anatomy, Abdomen and Pelvis, Pelvic Outlet." In *StatPearls* [*Internet*] . StatPearls Publishing, 2022.

13. Hemmerich, Andrea, Teresa Bandrowska, and Geneviève A. Dumas. "The Effects of Squatting While Pregnant on Pelvic Dimensions: A Computational Simulation to Understand Childbirth." *Journal of Biomechanics* 87 (2019): 64-74.

14. Borges, Margarida, Rita Moura, Dulce Oliveira, Marco Parente, Teresa Mascarenhas, and Renato Natal. "Effect of the Birthing Position on Its Evolution from a Biomechanical Point of View." *Computer Methods and Programs in Biomedicine* 200 (2021): 105921.

15. "FastStats - Births - Method of Delivery." Centers for Disease Control and Prevention, June 8, 2023. https://www.cdc.gov/nchs/fastats/delivery.htm.

16. Souka, A. P., T. Haritos, K. Basayiannis, N. Noikokyri, and A. Antsaklis. "Intrapartum Ultrasound for the Examination of the Fetal Head Position in Normal and Obstructed Labor." *The Journal of Maternal-Fetal & Neonatal Medicine* 13, no. 1 (2003): 59-63.

17. Vitner, D., Y. Paltieli, S. Haberman, R. Gonen, Y. Ville, and J. Nizard. "Prospective Multicenter Study of Ultrasound-Based Measurements of Fetal Head Station and Position Throughout Labor." *Ultrasound in Obstetrics & Gynecology* 46, no. 5 (2015): 611-615.

18. Frémondière, Pierre, and Estelle Servat. "Interval Versus External Pelvimetry: A Validation Study With Clinical Implications." *International Journal of Childbirth* (2023).

19. Wobser, Anna M., Zachary Adkins, and Randy W. Wobser. "Anatomy, Abdomen and Pelvis, Bones (Ilium, Ischium, and Pubis)." In *StatPearls* [*Internet*]. StatPearls Publishing, 2018.

CHAPTER 8

1. Trojner Bregar, Andreja, Miha Lucovnik, Ivan Verdenik, Franc Jager, Ksenija Gersak, and Robert E. Garfield. "Uterine Electromyography During Active Phase Compared with Latent Phase of Labor at Term." *Acta Obstetricia et Gynecologica Scandinavica* 95, no. 2 (2016): 197-202.

2. Hutchison, Julia, and Heba Mahdy. "Stages of Labor." In *StatPearls* [*Internet*]. StatPearls Publishing (2019).

3. Nelson, David B., James M. Alexander, Donald D. McIntire, and Kenneth J. Leveno. ""New or Not-So-New' Labor Management Practices and Cesarean Delivery for Arrest of Progress." *American Journal of Obstetrics and Gynecology* 222, no. 1 (2020): 71-e1.

4. Ridley, Renee T. "Diagnosis and Intervention for Occiput Posterior Malposition." *Journal of Obstetric, Gynecologic & Neonatal Nursing* 36, no. 2 (2007): 135-143.

5. Richmond, Anna K., and Janet R. Ashworth. "Management of Malposition and Malpresentation in Labour." *Obstetrics, Gynaecology & Reproductive Medicine* 33, no. 11 (2023): 325–333.

6. Michel, Sven CA, Annett Rake, Karl Treiber, Burkhardt Seifert, Rabih Chaoui, Renate Huch, Borut Marincek, and Rahel A. Kubik-Huch. "MR Obstetric Pelvimetry: Effect of Birthing Position on Pelvic Bony Dimensions." *American Journal of Roentgenology* 179, no. 4 (2002): 1063-1067.

7. Siccardi, Marco, Cristina Valle, and Fiorenza Di Matteo. "Dynamic External Pelvimetry Test in Third

Trimester Pregnant Women: Shifting Positions Affect Pelvic Biomechanics and Create More Room in Obstetric Diameters." *Cureus* 13, no. 3 (2021).

8. Berta, Marta, Helena Lindgren, Kyllike Christensson, Sollomon Mekonnen, and Mulat Adefris. "Effect of Maternal Birth Positions on Duration of Second Stage of Labor: Systematic Review and Meta-Analysis." *BMC Pregnancy and Childbirth* 19, no. 1 (2019): 1-8.

9. Roberts, Joyce, and Lisa Hanson. "Best Practices in Second Stage Labor Care: Maternal Bearing Down and Positioning." *Journal of Midwifery & Women's Health* 52, no. 3 (2007): 238-245.

10. Frémondière, Pierre, Lionel Thollon, François Marchal, and David Desseauve. "The Impact of Femoral Rotation on Sacroiliac Articulation During Pregnancy. Is There Evidence to Support Farabeuf's Hypothesis by Finite Element Modelization?" *European Journal of Obstetrics & Gynecology and Reproductive Biology* 290 (2023): 78-84.

11. American College of Nurse-Midwives; Midwives Alliance of North America; National Association of Certified Professional Midwives. "Supporting Healthy and Normal Physiologic Childbirth: A Consensus Statement by the American College of Nurse-Midwives, Midwives Alliance of North America, and the National Association of Certified Professional Midwives." *Journal of Midwifery & Women's Health* 57, no. 5 (2012): 529-532.

12. Begley, Cecily M., Gillian ML Gyte, Declan Devane, William McGuire, Andrew Weeks, and Linda M. Biesty. "Active Versus Expectant Management for Women in the Third Stage of Labour." *Cochrane Database of Systematic Reviews* 2 (2019).

13. Maisaroh, Siti, and Diani Maryani. "The Effectiveness of Counter Pressure and Endorphin Massage on Reducing Pain During First Stage of Labor in Intrapartum Mothers." In 8th International Conference on Public Health 2021, pp. 765-771. Sebelas Maret University, 2021.

14. Zuarez-Easton, Sivan, Offer Erez, Noah Zafran, Julia Carmeli, Gali Garmi, and Raed Salim. "Pharmacological and Non-Pharmacological Options for Pain Relief During Labor: An Expert Review." *American Journal of Obstetrics and Gynecology* (2023).

15. Shaban, Mona M. "Labor Pain Relief Using Transcutaneous Electrical Nerve Stimulation, Maternal and Fetal Impacts: A Randomized-Controlled Study." *Journal of Evidence-Based Women's Health Journal Society* 3, no. 4 (2013): 178-182.

CHAPTER 9

1. Selman, Rachel, Kate Early, Brianna Battles, Misty Seidenburg, Elizabeth Wendel, and Susan Westerlund. "Maximizing Recovery in the Postpartum Period: A Timeline for Rehabilitation from Pregnancy through Return to Sport." *International Journal of Sports Physical Therapy* 17, no. 6 (2022): 1170.

2. McCurdy, Ashley P., Normand G. Boulé, Allison Sivak, and Margie H. Davenport. "Effects of Exercise on Mild-to-Moderate Depressive Symptoms in the Postpartum Period: A Meta-Analysis." *Obstetrics & Gynecology* 129, no. 6 (2017): 1087-1097.

3. Torashima, Shizuka, Mina Samukawa, Kazumi Tsujino, and Yumi Sawada. "Postpartum as the Best Time for Physical Recovery and Health Care." *Journal of Novel Physiotherapy Rehabilitation* 7 (2023): 001-007.

4. Lee, Diane G., Linda-Joy Lee, and L. McLaughlin. "Stability, Continence and Breathing: The Role of Fascia Following Pregnancy and Delivery." *Journal of Bodywork and Movement Therapies* 12, no. 4 (2008): 333-348.

ACKNOWLEDGMENTS

THERE ARE SO MANY OF YOU who have supported me since the creation of Mamaste-Fit over the years—MamasteFit and this book are only possible due to the trust that many of you had in me in the early days. First, I need to thank my husband and father of my beautiful children, Barron. You are my biggest fan and hype man, and you truly supported and believed in me from the very beginning. Thank you to my oldest, Adeline, for being my inspiration to create MamasteFit. A hard birth for the both of us led me to support so many expectant families, not only in our community but across the world. Thank you to my littles, Eoghan, Sophie, and Zoe, for continuing to inspire me with each new birth and motherhood journey.

Thank you to my best friend and sister, Roxanne, for all that you do for MamasteFit as the cofounder. I could not (nor would I want to) do all that I do without you being a part of it.

Thank you to Casey for being my muse and the OG mama—from our first month postpartum trying to figure out a plan together, to creating our tribe in the prison gym of SPARTC, and expanding our reach across the globe, know that you are an important part of MamasteFit. And thank you to all the original MamasteFit mamas who trusted me in the infancy of MamasteFit and gave me the opportunity to learn and grow together as mothers.

Thank you to the MamasteFit team: Laura, Ashlie, Amanda, and Brittni! I truly appreciate all of your efforts at our gym and commitment to our moms—I could not do all the things I do without your support.

Thank you to Hayley and Johanna for sharing your pelvic floor expertise with me. The concepts you both have taught me expanded my understanding of the pelvis and positively affected my fitness programming.

And of course, thank you to my parents, Victor and Chong, for your support throughout my entire life and being the best grandparents to my kids. Everything I am and have been is thanks to your sacrifice and commitment to me and my siblings growing up.

ABOUT THE AUTHOR

GINA CONLEY holds an MS in Exercise Science and is the Founder/CEO of MamasteFit, an industry-leading perinatal fitness provider with a training facility located in Aberdeen, North Carolina. Aside from her work as a personal trainer specializing in perinatal fitness, Gina is a seasoned birth doula who has supported nearly 200 births in North Carolina. She is also a 7-year Army Veteran who served a combat tour to Afghanistan in support of Operations Enduring Freedom and Freedom Sentinel.

INDEX